QuickFACTS™

Lung CANCER

What You Need to Know—NOW

*Quick*FACTS™

From the Experts at the American Cancer Society

Lung
CANCER

What You Need to Know—NOW

Non–Small Cell Lung Cancer
Small Cell Lung Cancer

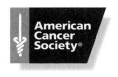

American
Cancer
Society®

Published by American Cancer Society /Health Promotions
1599 Clifton Road NE, Atlanta, Georgia 30329, USA

Copyright © 2007 American Cancer Society

Printed in the United States of America
Cover designed by Jill Dible, Atlanta, GA

5 4 3 2 1   07 08 09 10

Library of Congress Cataloging-in-Publication Data

Quick facts lung cancer : what you need to know--now /
From the Experts at the American Cancer Society.
    p. cm.
 Includes bibliographical references and index.
 ISBN-13: 978-0-944235-69-0 (pbk. : alk. paper)
 ISBN-10: 0-944235-69-7 (pbk. : alk. paper)
 1. Lungs--Cancer--Popular works. I. American Cancer
Society.

RC280.L8Q53 2007
616.99'424--dc22

                       2006016962

A Note to the Reader

This information represents the views of the doctors and nurses serving on the American Cancer Society's Cancer Information Database Editorial Board. These views are based on their interpretation of studies published in medical journals, as well as their own professional experience.

The treatment information in this book is not official policy of the Society and is not intended as medical advice to replace the expertise and judgment of your cancer care team. It is intended to help you and your family make informed decisions, together with your doctor.

Your doctor may have reasons for suggesting a treatment plan different from these general treatment options. Don't hesitate to ask him or her questions about your treatment options.

For more information, contact your American Cancer Society at 800-ACS-2345 or http://www.cancer.org

For special sales, contact us at **trade.sales@cancer.org**

Table of Contents

NON–SMALL CELL LUNG CANCER

SMALL CELL LUNG CANCER

Risk Factors and Causes

Prevention and Detection

Diagnosis and Staging

Questions To Ask

After Treatment

Latest Research

Resources

Your Non–Small Cell Lung Cancer

What Is Cancer?

Cancer* develops when **cells** in a part of the body begin to grow out of control. Although there are many kinds of cancer, they all start because of out-of-control growth of abnormal cells.

Normal body cells grow, divide, and die in an orderly fashion. During the early years of a person's life, normal cells divide more rapidly until the person becomes an adult. After that, cells in most parts of the body divide only to replace worn-out or dying cells and to repair injuries.

Because a **cancer cell** continues to grow and divide, it is different from a normal cell. Instead of dying, cancer cells outlive normal cells and continue to form new abnormal cells.

Cancer cells often travel to other parts of the body where they begin to grow and replace normal **tissue**. This process, called **metastasis**, occurs when the cancer cells get into the bloodstream or

*Terms in **bold type** are further explained in the dictionary that begins on page 175.*

lymphatic system of our body. However, when cells from a cancer like breast cancer spread to another organ like the liver, the cancer is still called breast cancer, not liver cancer.

Cancer cells develop because of damage to **DNA**. This substance is in every cell and directs all its activities. Most of the time when DNA becomes damaged the body is able to repair it. In cancer cells, the damaged DNA is not repaired. People can inherit damaged DNA, which accounts for inherited cancers. Many times though, a person's DNA becomes damaged by exposure to something in the environment, like smoking.

Cancer usually forms as a **tumor**. Some cancers, like leukemia, do not form tumors. Instead, these cancer cells involve the blood and blood-forming organs and circulate through other tissues where they grow.

Remember that not all tumors are cancerous. A **benign** (non-cancerous) **tumor** does not spread to other parts of the body (**metastasize**) and, with very rare exceptions, is not life-threatening.

Different types of cancer can behave very differently. For example, lung cancer and breast cancer are very different diseases. They grow at different rates and respond to different treatments. That is why people with cancer need treatment that is aimed at their particular kind of cancer.

Cancer is the second leading cause of death in the United States. Nearly half of all men and a little over one-third of all women in the United States will develop cancer during their lifetimes. Today, millions of people are living with cancer or have had cancer. The risk of developing most types of cancer can be reduced by changes in a person's lifestyle, for example, by quitting smoking and eating a better diet. The sooner a cancer is found and treatment begins, the better a patient's chances of living for many years.

What Is Non–Small Cell Lung Cancer?

Note: This section is specifically for the non–small cell type of lung cancer. The treatment for each type of lung cancer (small cell vs. non–small cell) is very different. So the information for one type will not apply to the other type. If you are not sure which type of lung cancer you have, it is very important to ask your doctor so you can be sure the information you receive is correct.

The Lungs

Your lungs are 2 sponge-like organs found in your chest. Your right lung is divided into 3 sections, called lobes. Your left lung has 2 lobes. It is smaller because your heart takes up more room on that side of the body. When you breathe, air goes into your lungs through the **trachea** (windpipe). The trachea divides into tubes called the **bronchi**, which divide into smaller branches called the **bronchioles**. At the end of the bronchioles are tiny air sacs known as **alveoli**. Many tiny blood vessels run through the alveoli, absorbing oxygen from the inhaled air into your bloodstream and

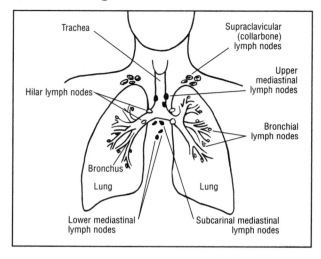

Trachea

Supraclavicular (collarbone) lymph nodes

Upper mediastinal lymph nodes

Hilar lymph nodes

Bronchial lymph nodes

Bronchus

Lung

Lung

Lower mediastinal lymph nodes

Subcarinal mediastinal lymph nodes

releasing carbon dioxide. Taking in oxygen and getting rid of carbon dioxide are your lungs' main functions. A lining, called the **pleura**, surrounds the lungs. This slippery lining protects your lungs and helps them slide back and forth as they expand and contract during breathing.

Most lung cancers start in the lining of the bronchi, but they can also begin in other areas such as the trachea, bronchioles, or alveoli. Lung cancers are thought to develop over a period of many years. First, there may be areas of **precancerous** changes in the lung. These changes do not form a mass or tumor. They cannot be seen on an **x-ray** and they do not cause **symptoms**. But these precancerous changes can be found by analyzing cells in the lining of the airways of smoke-damaged lungs.

Recently, molecular abnormalities believed to be precancerous have been identified in cells from people at **high risk** to develop lung cancers (for example, survivors from one prior lung cancer). These precancerous changes often progress to true cancer. As a cancer develops, the cancer cells may produce chemicals that cause new blood vessels to form nearby. These new blood vessels nourish the cancer cells, which can continue to grow and form a tumor large enough to be seen on x-rays. Cells from the cancer can break away from the original tumor and spread to other parts of the body. As noted earlier, this process is called metastasis. Lung cancer is a life-threatening disease because it often spreads in this way even before it can be detected on a chest x-ray.

One of the ways lung cancer can spread is through the lymphatic system. Lymphatic vessels are similar to veins but carry lymph instead of blood. Lymph is a clear fluid that contains tissue waste products and **immune system** cells. Lymphatic vessels of the lungs lead to nearby **lymph nodes** inside the chest. These nodes are located around the bronchi and in the **mediastinum** (the area between the 2 lungs). Cancer cells may enter lymph vessels and spread out along these vessels to reach lymph nodes. Lymph nodes are small, bean-shaped collections of immune system cells that are important in fighting infections. When lung cancer cells reach the lymph nodes, they can continue to grow. If cancer cells have multiplied in the lymph nodes, they are more likely to have spread to other organs of the body as well. **Staging** of the cancer and decisions about lung cancer treatment are based on whether the cancer has spread to the nearby lymph nodes in the mediastinum. These topics are discussed later in this book.

Types of Lung Cancer

There are 2 major types of lung cancer:

- small cell lung cancer (SCLC)
- non–small cell lung cancer (NSCLC)

If a lung cancer has characteristics of both types it is called a mixed small cell/large cell **carcinoma**. This is uncommon. These 2 types of lung cancer are discussed separately because they are treated very differently.

Non–Small Cell Lung Cancer

About 85%–90% of lung cancers are non–small cell (NSCLC). There are 3 subtypes of NSCLC. The cells in these subtypes differ in size, shape, and chemical makeup when looked at under a microscope.

- **squamous cell carcinoma:** About 25%–30% of all lung cancers are squamous cell carcinomas. They are linked to a history of smoking and tend to be found centrally, near the bronchi.

- **adenocarcinoma:** This type accounts for about 40% of lung cancers. It is usually found in the outer region of the lung. People with bronchioloalveolar adenocarcinoma (sometimes called bronchioalveolar carcinoma) tend to have a better outlook **(prognosis)** than those with other types of lung cancer.
- **large-cell undifferentiated carcinoma:** This type of cancer accounts for about 10%–15% of lung cancers. It may appear in any part of the lung, and it tends to grow and spread quickly, resulting in a poor prognosis.

Other Types of Lung Cancer

In addition to the 2 main types of lung cancer, other tumors can occur in the lungs. Some of these are noncancerous (benign). **Carcinoid tumors** of the lung account for fewer than 5% of lung tumors. Most are slow-growing tumors that are called typical carcinoid tumors. They are generally cured by surgery. Although some typical carcinoid tumors can spread, they usually have a better prognosis (outlook) than small cell or non– small cell lung cancer. **Atypical** carcinoid tumors are much less common than typical carcinoids, but they are more likely to grow and spread quickly.

Cancer that has spread to the lungs from other organs (such as the breast, pancreas, kidney, or skin) is called **metastatic** cancer. Treatment for metastatic cancer to the lungs depends on where it started (the **primary site**).

What Are the Key Statistics About Lung Cancer?

During 2007, there will be about 213,380 new cases of lung cancer (both small cell and non–small cell), 114,760 among men and 98,620 among women. Lung cancer will account for about 15% of all new cancers. Lung cancer mainly occurs in the elderly. Nearly 70% of people diagnosed with lung cancer are older than 65; fewer than 3% of all cases are found in people under the age of 45. The chance that a man will develop lung cancer is 1 in 12, and for a woman, it is 1 in 16. This figure includes all people and doesn't take into account whether or not they smoke.

Lung cancer is the leading cause of cancer death among both men and women. There will be an estimated 160,390 deaths from lung cancer (89,510 among men and 70,880 among women) in 2007, accounting for around 29% of all cancer deaths. More people die of lung cancer than of colon, breast, and prostate cancers combined. Despite the very serious prognosis of lung cancer, some people are cured and there are currently about 330,000 long-term survivors.

Nearly 60% of people diagnosed with either type of lung cancer die within 1 year of their diagnosis. Nearly 75% die within 2 years. This has not improved in 10 years. Only about 16% of people diagnosed with non–small cell lung cancer survive this disease after 5 years.

Black men are about 50% more likely to develop non–small cell lung cancer than white men. Both black and white women have a lower rate, with the rate being slightly higher in black women. The rate of non–small cell lung cancer is dropping rapidly in men and much more slowly in women.

Risk Factors and Causes

What Are the Risk Factors for Non–Small Cell Lung Cancer?

A **risk factor** is anything that increases your chance of getting a disease such as cancer. Different cancers have different risk factors. For example, unprotected exposure to strong sunlight is a risk factor for skin cancer. Several risk factors can make you more likely to develop lung cancer:

Tobacco Smoking

Smoking is by far the leading risk factor for lung cancer. At the beginning of the 20th century, lung cancer was a rare disease. The introduction of manufactured cigarettes, which made them readily available, changed this. About 87% of lung cancers are thought to result from smoking and some of the rest from passive exposure to tobacco smoke. The longer you smoke and the more packs per day you smoke, the greater your risk.

If you stop smoking before a cancer develops, your damaged lung tissue gradually starts to return to normal. Ten years after stopping smoking, your risk is reduced to one-third of what it would have been if you continued to smoke. Cigar smoking and pipe smoking are almost as likely to cause lung cancer as cigarette smoking. There is no evidence that smoking low tar or "light" cigarettes reduces the risk of lung cancer. There is concern that mentholated cigarettes may increase the risk. It is thought that the menthol may allow smokers to inhale more deeply.

If you don't smoke, but breathe in the smoke of others (called secondhand smoke or environmental tobacco smoke), you are also at increased risk for lung cancer. A nonsmoker who is married to a smoker has a 30% greater risk of developing lung cancer than the spouse of a nonsmoker. Workers who have been exposed to tobacco smoke in the workplace are also more likely to get lung cancer.

Hookah smoking has become popular among young people. It is actively marketed as safer than cigarettes because the percentage of tobacco in the product smoked is low and the smoke is filtered through water. However, experts at the American Cancer Society believe that smoking any amount of tobacco is dangerous. Studies have shown that hookah smoke contains the same cancer-causing substances as cigarettes. It is addictive and may lead to cigarette smoking in the future.

Arsenic

High levels of arsenic in drinking water may increase the risk of lung cancer. This is even more pronounced in smokers.

Asbestos

If you are an asbestos worker, you are about 7 times more likely to die of lung cancer. Exposure to asbestos fibers is an important risk factor for lung cancer. And if you are or have been an asbestos worker who smokes, your lung cancer risk is 50 to 90 times greater than that of people in general. Both smokers and nonsmokers exposed to asbestos also have a greater risk of developing a type of cancer that starts from the pleura (the layer of cells that line the outer surface of the lung). This cancer is called mesothelioma.

In recent years, government regulations have nearly stopped the use of asbestos in commercial and industrial products. It is still present in many homes and commercial buildings but is not considered harmful as long as it is not released into the air by deterioration, demolition, or renovation.

Radon

When uranium breaks down naturally it produces radon, a radioactive gas that cannot be seen, tasted, or smelled. Outdoors, there is so little radon that it is not dangerous. But indoors, radon can be more concentrated and become a possible risk for cancer. Recently, concerns have been raised about houses in some parts of the United States built over soil with natural uranium deposits that can create high indoor radon levels. Studies from these areas have found that the risk of lung cancer may double or even triple if you have lived for many years in a radon-contaminated house. This is a very small increase though, when it is compared to the lung cancer risk from tobacco.

Smokers are especially sensitive to the effects of radon. State and local offices of the Environmental Protection Agency can give you the names of reliable companies that perform radon testing and renovation.

Cancer-Causing Agents in the Workplace

There are other **carcinogens** (cancer-causing agents) found in the workplace that can increase your lung cancer risk:

- radioactive ores such as uranium
- inhaled chemicals or minerals such as arsenic, beryllium, vinyl chloride, nickel chromates, coal products, mustard gas, and chloromethyl ethers
- fuels such as gasoline
- diesel exhaust

The government and industry have taken major steps in recent years to protect workers. But the dangers are still present, and if you work around these agents, you should be very careful to avoid exposure.

Marijuana

More tar is contained in marijuana than in cigarettes. Marijuana is also inhaled very deeply and the smoke is held in the lungs for a long time. Marijuana is smoked all the way to the end where tar content is the highest. Many of the cancer-causing substances in tobacco are also found in marijuana. Because marijuana is an illegal substance, it is not possible to control whether it contains pesticides and other additives. Medical reports suggest marijuana may cause cancers of the mouth and throat.

It has been hard to prove a connection between marijuana and lung cancer because it is not easy to gather information about the use of illegal drugs. Also, many marijuana smokers also smoke cigarettes. This makes it difficult to know how much of the risk is from tobacco and how much is from marijuana.

Radiation Therapy to the Lungs

People who have had **radiation therapy** to the chest for cancer are at higher risk for lung cancer, particularly if they smoke. Typical patients are those treated for **Hodgkin disease** or women who receive radiation to the chest after a mastectomy for breast cancer. Women who receive radiation therapy to the breast after a lumpectomy do not have a higher than expected risk of lung cancer. But if they smoke, their chance of lung cancer goes up markedly.

Talc and Talcum Powder

In the past, some studies suggested that talc miners and millers have a higher risk of lung cancer and other respiratory diseases because of their exposure to industrial grade talc. Recent studies of talc miners have not found an increase in lung cancer rate. Talcum powder is made from talc, a mineral that in its natural form may contain asbestos. By law since 1973, all home-use talcum products (baby, body, and facial powders) have been asbestos-free.

The use of cosmetic talcum powder has not been found to increase your risk of lung cancer.

Other Mineral Exposures

People with silicosis and berylliosis (lung diseases caused by breathing in certain minerals) also have a higher risk of lung cancer.

Personal and Family History of Lung Cancer

If you have had lung cancer, you have a higher risk of developing another lung cancer. Brothers, sisters, and children of those who have had lung cancer may have a slightly higher risk of lung cancer themselves. Recently, a group called the Genetic Epidemiology of Lung Cancer Consortium studied families with a strong history of lung cancer. They found that the susceptibility to lung cancer might reside on a particular **chromosome** (chromosome 6). People who have the abnormality on chromosome 6 will more readily develop lung cancer even if they only smoke a little. Other family members who lack the genetic abnormality have to smoke more to develop lung cancer.

Another study, conducted in Iceland, found that if a person's **first degree relative** (sibling, parent) had lung cancer, that person's chance of developing the disease doubles. Although smoking played a role, in this study, the family members didn't smoke any more than non-family members. Other studies have shown that the risk of lung cancer increases in a family if someone in the family developed the cancer at a young age.

Diet

Some reports have indicated that a diet low in fruits and vegetables may increase the chances of getting cancer if you are exposed to tobacco smoke. Evidence is growing that fruits and vegetables may protect you against lung cancer.

Air Pollution

In some cities, air pollution can slightly increase the risk of lung cancer. This risk is far less than that caused by smoking.

Do We Know What Causes Non–Small Cell Lung Cancer?

Tobacco smoking is by far the leading cause of lung cancer. More than 87% of lung cancers are caused directly by smoking, and some of the rest are caused by environmental exposure to tobacco smoke. Other risk factors for lung cancer include a family or personal history of lung cancer and exposure to cancer-causing agents in the workplace or the environment.

Recently, scientists have begun to understand how these risk factors produce certain changes in the DNA of cells in the lungs, causing them to grow abnormally and form cancers. DNA is the genetic material that carries the instructions for nearly everything our cells do. We usually resemble our parents because they passed their DNA on to us. However, DNA affects more than our outward appearance. Some genes (parts of our DNA) contain instructions for controlling when cells grow and divide.

Genes that promote cell division are called **oncogenes**. Genes that slow down cell division or cause cells to die at the appropriate time are called **tumor suppressor genes**.

It is known that cancer can be caused by a DNA **mutation** (defect) that activates (turns on) oncogenes or inactivates (turns off) tumor suppressor genes. Some people inherit DNA mutations from their parents that greatly increase their risk for developing breast, ovarian, colorectal, and several other cancers. However, inherited oncogene or tumor suppressor gene mutations are not believed to cause very many lung cancers.

Oncogene and tumor suppressor gene mutations related to lung cancer usually develop during life rather than before birth as an inherited mutation. Every time a cell prepares to divide into 2 new cells, it must duplicate its DNA. This process is not perfect and copying errors occur.

Fortunately, cells have repair enzymes that proofread the DNA, but some errors may slip past. Some people may have faulty DNA repair mechanisms that make them especially vulnerable to cancer-causing chemicals and radiation. Acquired mutations in lung cells often result from exposure to cancer-causing chemicals in tobacco smoke. Acquired changes in genes, such as the *p53* tumor suppressor gene and the *ras* oncogene, are thought to be important in the development of lung cancer. Changes in these and similar genes may also make some lung cancers likely to grow and invade more rapidly than others.

Although inherited mutations of oncogenes or tumor suppressor genes rarely cause lung cancers, some people seem to inherit a reduced ability to detoxify (break down) certain types of cancer-causing chemicals.

Other people may inherit an increased tendency to activate carcinogens, making these genes even more dangerous. These people are more sensitive to the cancer-causing effects of tobacco smoke and certain industrial chemicals. Researchers are developing tests that may help identify such people, but these tests are not yet reliable enough for routine use. Therefore, doctors recommend that all people avoid tobacco smoke and hazardous industrial chemicals.

Prevention and Detection

Can Non–Small Cell Lung Cancer Be Prevented?

The best way to prevent lung cancer is to not smoke and to avoid breathing in other people's smoke. If you already smoke, you should quit. You should also avoid breathing in other people's smoke. Likewise, working and living in an environment free of cancer-causing chemicals will also be helpful. A healthy diet with lots of fruits and vegetables may also help prevent this cancer.

There have been many attempts to reduce the risk of lung cancer in current or former smokers by giving them high doses of vitamins or vitamin-like drugs. These have been completely unsuccessful. In one study, a nutrient related to vitamin A called *beta-carotene* appeared to increase the rate of cancer.

Some people who get lung cancer do not have any apparent risk factors. Although we know how to prevent most lung cancers, at this time we don't know how to prevent all of them.

Can Non–Small Cell Lung Cancer Be Found Early?

Usually symptoms of lung cancer do not appear until the disease is in an **advanced stage**. But some lung cancers are diagnosed early because they are found as a result of tests for other medical conditions. For example, a diagnosis may be made by an **imaging test** or **scan** (such as a chest x-ray or chest **CT scan**), **bronchoscopy** (viewing the inside of bronchi through a flexible lighted tube), or **sputum cytology** (microscopic examination of cells in coughed up phlegm) performed for other reasons in patients with heart disease, pneumonia, or other lung conditions.

Screening Tests for Lung Cancer

Screening is the use of tests or examinations to detect a disease in people without symptoms of that disease. For example, the Pap test is used to screen for cervical cancer. Because lung cancer usually spreads beyond the lungs before causing any symptoms, an effective screening program to detect lung cancer early could save many lives.

Thus far, no lung cancer screening test has been shown to prevent people from dying of this disease. The use of chest x-rays and sputum cytology (checking phlegm under the microscope to find cancer cells) has been tested for several years. The studies, which have been recently updated, have concluded that these tests could not find many lung cancers early enough to improve a person's chance for a cure. For this reason, lung cancer screening is not a routine practice for the general public or even for people at increased risk, such as smokers.

Recently, a new x-ray technique called spiral or helical low-dose CT scanning has been successful in detecting early lung cancer in smokers and former smokers. But it has not yet been shown whether this technique will lower the chances of dying from lung cancer. One major problem with this test is that it finds a lot of abnormalities that turn out to not be cancer. This leads to a lot of unnecessary testing and even surgery.

A large **clinical trial** called the National Lung Screening Trial (NLST) is testing whether spiral CT scanning of people at high risk of lung cancer will save lives. This trial, which began in 2002, has studied about 50,000 people. It is now closed to new subjects. Soon we will learn whether spiral CT scanning will catch lung cancer early enough to save lives. Until this information is available, people who are interested in testing should understand the limits and benefits of low-dose CT scanning.

The United States Preventive Services Task Force, a group of experts gathered together by the U.S. government, recently concluded that no one has shown that screening for lung cancer helps patients. Their statement:

"The USPSTF recommends neither for nor against using chest x-ray, computed tomography (CT scan), or sputum cytologic examination to look for lung cancer in people who have no symptoms to suggest the disease. If screening is being considered, doctors and patients should discuss the pros and cons of screening before going ahead with x-ray, CT scan, or sputum cytologic examination to screen for lung cancer. Patients should be aware that there are no studies showing that screening helps people live longer. They should also know that **false-positive** test results are common and can lead to unnecessary worry, testing, and surgery."

People who are current smokers also should realize that the best way to avoid dying of lung cancer is to stop smoking. This is the surest route to good health.

The American Cancer Society recommends that, as much as possible, people who were smokers, are current smokers, have been exposed to secondhand smoke, or have worked around materials that increase the risk for lung cancer, be aware of their continuing lung cancer risk. These individuals should talk with their doctors about their likelihood of developing lung cancer and about the potential benefits and risks of lung cancer screening. The most obvious potential benefit is detection of some lung cancers at an early stage. Some studies have shown that CT scans can find lung cancer when most cases are curable. The main risk is that many of the scans will produce inconclusive findings that will need to be resolved by further tests that are invasive, uncomfortable, expensive, and have side effects that can be serious and even fatal. After a discussion about what is and is not known about the value of testing for early lung cancer detection, if you and your doctor decide in favor of testing, then be sure to choose an institution that has experience in lung scanning and that supports a multidisciplinary program dedicated to evaluation of high-risk individuals.

Diagnosis and Staging

How Is Non–Small Cell Lung Cancer Diagnosed?

If there is a reason to suspect you may have lung cancer, your doctor will use one or more methods to find out if the disease is really present. In addition, a **biopsy** of the lung tissue can confirm the **diagnosis** of cancer and also give valuable information that will help in making treatment decisions. If these tests find lung cancer, more tests will be done to find out how far the cancer has spread.

Common Signs and Symptoms of Lung Cancer

Although most lung cancers do not cause any symptoms until they have spread too far to be cured, symptoms do occur in some people with early lung cancer. If you go to your doctor when you first notice symptoms, your cancer might be diagnosed and treated while it is in a curable stage. Or, at the least, you could live longer with a better **quality of life**. These are the most common symptoms of lung cancer:

- a cough that does not go away
- chest pain, often aggravated by deep breathing, coughing, and even laughing

- hoarseness
- weight loss and loss of appetite
- bloody or rust-colored sputum (spit or phlegm)
- shortness of breath
- recurring infections such as bronchitis and pneumonia
- new onset of wheezing

When lung cancer spreads to distant organs, it may cause these effects:
- bone pain
- neurologic changes (such as headache, weakness or numbness of a limb, dizziness, or recent onset of a seizure)
- jaundice (yellow coloring of the skin and eyes)
- masses near the surface of the body, due to cancer spreading to the skin or to lymph nodes (collections of immune system cells) in the neck or above the collarbone

If you have any of these problems, see your doctor right away. These symptoms could be the first warning of a lung cancer. Many of these symptoms can also result from other causes or from noncancerous diseases of the lungs, heart, and other organs. Seeing a doctor is the only way to find out. Other symptoms are listed below.

Horner syndrome
Cancer of the upper part of the lungs may damage a nerve that passes from the upper chest into

your neck. Doctors sometimes call these cancers Pancoast tumors. Their most common symptom is severe shoulder pain. Sometimes they also cause Horner syndrome. Horner syndrome is the medical name for the group of symptoms consisting of drooping or weakness of one eyelid, reduced or absent perspiration on the same side of your face, and a smaller pupil (dark part in the center of the eye) on that side.

Paraneoplastic syndromes

Some lung cancers may produce **hormone**-like or other substances that enter the bloodstream and cause problems with distant tissues and organs, even though the cancer has not spread to those tissues or organs. These problems are called paraneoplastic (Latin for "tumor-related") syndromes. Sometimes these syndromes may be the first symptoms of early lung cancer. Because the symptoms affect other organs, patients and their doctors may suspect at first that diseases other than lung cancer are causing them.

These are the most common paraneoplastic syndromes caused by non–small cell lung cancer:

- Hypercalcemia (high blood calcium levels), causing urinary frequency, constipation, weakness, dizziness, confusion, and other nervous system problems.
- Excess growth (sometimes painful) of certain bones, especially those in the finger tips. The medical term for this is hypertrophic osteoarthropathy.

- Production of substances that activate the clotting system, leading to blood clots.
- Excess breast growth in men. The medical term for this condition is gynecomastia.

Medical History and Physical Exam

Your doctor will take a medical history (health-related interview) to check for risk factors and symptoms. Your doctor will also examine you to look for signs of lung cancer and other health problems.

Imaging Tests

Imaging tests use x-rays, magnetic fields, or radioactive substances to create pictures of the inside of your body. Several imaging tests are used to find lung cancer and determine where it may have spread in the body.

Chest x-ray

This is the first test your doctor will order to look for any mass or spot on the lungs. It is a plain x-ray of your chest and can be done in any outpatient setting. If the x-ray is normal, you probably don't have lung cancer. If something suspicious is seen, your doctor may order additional tests.

Computed tomography

Computed tomography (CT) is an x-ray procedure that produces detailed cross-sectional images of your body. Instead of taking one picture, as does a conventional x-ray, a CT scanner takes many pictures as it rotates around you. A computer then combines these pictures into an image of a slice of your body. The machine will take pictures and form multiple images of the part of your body that is being studied. Often after the first set of pictures is taken you will receive an **intravenous** injection of a "dye" or radiocontrast agent that helps better outline structures in your body. A second set of pictures is then taken.

CT scans take longer than regular x-rays and you will need to lie still on a table while they are being done. But just like other computerized devices, they are getting faster and your stay might be pleasantly short. The newest CT scans take only seconds to complete. Also, you might feel a bit confined by the ring-like equipment you're in when the pictures are being taken.

The contrast "dye" is injected through an IV line. Some people are allergic to the dye and get hives, a flushed feeling, or, rarely, more serious reactions like trouble breathing and low blood pressure. Be sure to tell your doctor if you have ever had a reaction to any contrast material used for x-rays. If you have, you may need medicine before you can have such an injection during your test.

You may also be asked to drink a contrast solution. This helps outline your intestine if your doctor is looking at organs in your abdomen to see if the lung cancer has spread.

The CT scan will provide precise information about the size, shape, and position of a tumor and can help find enlarged lymph nodes that might contain cancer that has spread from the lung. CT scans are more sensitive than a routine chest x-ray in finding early lung cancers. This test is also used to find masses in the adrenal glands, brain, and other internal organs that may be affected by the spread of lung cancer.

Magnetic resonance imaging

Magnetic resonance imaging (MRI) uses radio waves and strong magnets instead of x-rays. The energy from the radio waves is absorbed and then released in a pattern formed by the type of tissue and by certain diseases. A computer translates the pattern of radio waves given off by the tissues into a very detailed image of parts of the body. Not only does this produce cross-sectional slices of the body like a CT scanner, it can also produce slices that are parallel with the length of your body.

A contrast material might be injected just as with CT scans, but is used less often. MRI scans take longer—often up to an hour. Also, you have to be placed inside a tube-like piece of equipment, which is confining and can upset people with claustrophobia. The machine makes a thumping noise that you may find annoying. Some places will provide headphones with music to block this out. MRI images are particularly useful in detecting lung cancer that has spread to the brain or spinal cord.

Positron emission tomography

Positron emission tomography (PET) uses glucose (a form of sugar) that contains a radioactive atom. A small amount of the radioactive material is injected into a vein. Cancer cells in the body absorb large amounts of the radioactive sugar and a special camera can detect the radioactivity. This can be a very important test if you have early-stage lung cancer. Your doctor will use this test to see if the cancer has spread to lymph nodes. It is also helpful in telling whether a shadow on your chest x-ray is cancer. A **PET scan** is also useful when your doctor thinks the cancer has spread, but doesn't know where. PET scans can be used instead of several different x-rays because they scan your whole body. Newer devices combine a CT scan and a PET scan to better pinpoint the tumor.

Bone scans

In a bone scan, a small amount of radioactive substance (usually technetium diphosphonate) is injected into a vein. The amount of radioactivity used is very low and causes no long-term effects. This substance builds up in areas of bone that may be abnormal because of cancer metastasis. Areas of diseased bone will be seen on the bone scan image as dense, gray to black areas, called "hot spots." These areas may suggest the presence of metastatic cancer, but arthritis, infection, or other bone diseases can also cause a similar pattern. Bone scans are routinely done in patients with small cell lung cancer. Usually, they are only done in patients with non–small cell lung cancer when other test results or symptoms suggest that the cancer has spread to the bones.

Procedures That Sample Tissues and Cells

One or more of these tests will be used to confirm that a lung mass seen on imaging tests is, indeed, lung cancer. These tests collect cells from the suspicious area and are also used to determine the exact type of lung cancer you may have and to help determine how far it may have spread. A **pathologist**, a doctor who specializes in laboratory tests to diagnose diseases such as cancer, will examine the cells using a microscope. If you have any questions about your pathology results or any diagnostic tests, do not hesitate to ask your doctor. You can get a second opinion of your pathology report, called a pathology review, by having your tissue specimen sent to another laboratory recommended by your doctor.

Sputum cytology

A sample of phlegm (mucus you cough up from the lungs) is examined under a microscope to see if cancer cells are present. The best way to do this is to get early morning samples from you 3 days in a row.

Needle biopsy

A needle can be guided into the suspicious area while your lungs are being looked at with fluoroscopy (fluoroscopy is like an x-ray, but the image is shown on a screen rather than on film). CT scans can also be used to guide the placement of needles. Unlike fluoroscopy, CT doesn't provide a continuous picture, so the needle is inserted in the direction of the mass, a CT image is taken, and the direction of the needle is guided based on the image. This process is repeated a few times until the CT image confirms that the needle is within the mass. A tiny sample of the target area is sucked into a syringe and examined under the microscope to see if cancer cells are present.

A thin needle can also be inserted through the wall of the trachea to sample nearby lymph nodes by using a flexible, lighted tube called a broncho-scope. This procedure, called **transtracheal fine needle aspiration**, is often used to take samples of subcarinal lymph nodes (around the point where the windpipe branches into the left and right bronchi) and mediastinal lymph nodes (along the windpipe and the major bronchial tube areas). (See illustration, page 4.)

Bronchoscopy

You will need to be sedated for this exam. A bronchoscope is passed through your mouth into the bronchi (the larger tubes which carry air to the lungs). This can help find some tumors or blockages in the lungs. At the same time, it can also be used in performing a biopsy (taking samples of tissue) or taking samples of lung secretions to be examined under a microscope for cancer cells or precancerous cells. Studies are being done to see if annual exams will be helpful in finding **premalignant** changes in people at high risk.

Endobronchial ultrasound

In this bronchoscopy technique, the broncho-scope is fitted with an **ultrasound** emitter and receiver at its tip. This may be helpful in gauging the size of the tumor and in spotting enlarged lymph nodes. A fine needle passed through the biopsy channel can sample these nodes under ultrasound guidance.

Endoscopic esophageal ultrasound

In **endoscopic esophageal ultrasound (EUS)**, the bronchoscope is fitted with an ultrasound emitter and receiver at its tip and passed into the esophagus. This is done with light sedation. The esophagus is close to some lymph nodes inside the chest, and lung cancer can spread to these lymph nodes. Ultrasound images taken from inside the esophagus can be helpful in finding large lymph nodes inside the chest that might contain metastatic lung cancer. A fine needle passed through a channel on the scope can sample these nodes under ultrasound guidance.

Mediastinoscopy and mediastinotomy

For both of these procedures, you will receive general **anesthesia** (be put into a deep sleep). With **mediastinoscopy** a small cut is made in your neck and a hollow lighted tube is inserted behind the sternum (breastbone). Special instruments, operated through this tube, can be used to take a tissue sample from the mediastinal lymph nodes (along the windpipe and the major bronchial tube areas). Looking at the samples under a microscope can show whether cancer cells are present.

With **mediastinotomy**, the surgeon removes samples of mediastinal lymph nodes while the patient is under general anesthesia. Unlike mediastinoscopy, with mediastinotomy the surgeon opens the chest cavity by making a small incision beside the sternum. This allows the surgeon to reach lymph nodes that are not reached by standard mediastinoscopy.

Thoracentesis and thoracoscopy

Thoracentesis and **thoracoscopy** are done to find out whether a buildup of fluid around the lungs (pleural effusion) is the result of cancer spreading to the membranes that cover the lungs (pleura). The buildup might also be caused by a condition such as heart failure or an infection.

For thoracentesis, the skin is numbed and a needle is placed between the ribs to drain the fluid. The fluid is checked under a microscope to look for cancer cells. Chemical tests of the fluid are also sometimes useful in distinguishing a **malignant** (cancerous) pleural effusion from a benign one. Once malignant pleural fluid has been diagnosed, thoracentesis may be repeated to remove more fluid. Fluid buildup can prevent the lungs from filling with air, so thoracentesis can help the patient breathe better.

Thoracoscopy is a procedure that uses a thin, lighted tube connected to a video camera and monitor to view the space between the lungs and the chest wall. Using this, the doctor can see cancer deposits and remove a small piece of the tissue to be examined under the microscope. Thoracoscopy can also be used to sample lymph nodes and fluid.

Blood counts and blood chemistry

A complete **blood count** (CBC) determines whether your blood has the correct number of various cell types. For example, it can show if you have anemia. This test will be repeated regularly if you are treated with **chemotherapy**, because these drugs temporarily affect blood-forming cells of the bone marrow. The blood chemistry tests can spot abnormalities in some of your organs. If cancer has spread to the liver and bones, it may cause certain chemical abnormalities in the blood. If one of these in particular, called the LDH, is elevated, it usually means that the outlook for cure or long-term survival isn't as good.

How Is Non–Small Cell Lung Cancer Staged?

Staging is the process of finding out whether your cancer is localized or widespread. It describes how far the cancer has spread. Your treatment and prognosis (the outlook for chances of survival) depend, to a large extent, on the cancer's stage. The many tests just described are used to stage the cancer.

Staging of Non–Small Cell Lung Cancer

The system used to describe the growth and spread of non–small cell lung cancer (NSCLC) is the **TNM staging system**, also known as the **American Joint Committee on Cancer (AJCC) staging system**. **T** stands for tumor (its size and how far it has spread within the lung and to nearby organs), **N** stands for spread to lymph **n**odes, and **M** is for **m**etastasis (spread to distant organs). In TNM staging, information about the tumor, lymph nodes, and metastasis is combined and a stage is assigned to specific TNM groupings. The grouped stages are described using the number 0 and Roman numerals from I to IV (1 to 4). Some stages are subdivided into A and B.

Non–Small Cell Lung Cancer T Categories

T categories are based on the lung cancer's size, its spread and location within the lungs, and its spread to nearby tissues.

Tis

Cancer is found only in the layer of cells lining the air passages. It has not invaded other lung tissues. This stage is also known as **carcinoma in situ**.

T1

The cancer is no larger than 3 cm (slightly less than 1¼ inches), has not spread to the membranes that surround the lungs (visceral pleura), and does not affect the main branches of the bronchi.

T2

The cancer has one or more of the following features:

- It is larger than 3 cm.
- It involves a main bronchus, but is not closer than 2 cm (about ¾ inch) to the point where the windpipe (trachea) branches into the left and right main bronchi (carina).
- It has spread to the membranes that surround the lungs (pleura).
- The cancer may partially clog the airways, but this has not caused the entire lung to collapse or develop pneumonia.

T3

The cancer has one or more of the following features:

- Spread to the chest wall, the breathing muscle that separates the chest from the abdomen (diaphragm), the membranes surrounding the space between the 2 lungs (mediastinal pleura), or membranes of the sac surrounding the heart (parietal pericardium).
- Invades a main bronchus and is closer than 2 cm (about ¾ inch) to the point where the windpipe (trachea) branches into the left and right main bronchi (carina), but does not affect this area.
- Has grown into the airways enough to cause an entire lung to collapse or to cause pneumonia in the entire lung.

T4

The cancer has one or more of the following features:

- Spread to the space behind the chest bone and in front of the heart (mediastinum), the heart, the windpipe (trachea), the esophagus (tube connecting the throat to the stomach), the backbone, or the point where the windpipe branches into the left and right main bronchi (carina).
- Two or more separate tumor nodules are present in the same lobe.

- There is a fluid containing cancer cells in the space surrounding the lung (a malignant pleural effusion).

Non–Small Cell Lung Cancer N Categories

The N category depends on which, if any, of the lymph nodes near the lungs are affected by the cancer.

N0

No spread to lymph nodes.

N1

Spread to lymph nodes within the lung and/or located around the area where the bronchus enters the lung (hilar lymph nodes). Metastases affect lymph nodes only on the same side as the cancerous lung.

N2

Spread to lymph nodes around the point where the windpipe branches into the left and right bronchi (subcarinal lymph nodes) or in the space behind the chest bone and in front of the heart (mediastinum). Affected lymph nodes are on the same side of the cancerous lung.

N3

Spread to lymph nodes near the collarbone on either side, and/or to hilar or mediastinal lymph nodes on the side opposite the cancerous lung.

Non–Small Cell Lung Cancer M Categories

The M category depends on whether the cancer has spread to any distant tissues and organs.

M0

No spread to distant organs or areas. Sites considered distant include other lobes of the lungs, lymph nodes beyond those mentioned in N stages, and other organs or tissues such as the liver, bones, or brain.

M1

The cancer has spread to one or more distant sites. This can be to another organ or to the other lung or a different lobe of the same lung. This also refers to a second tumor arising in a different part of the lung, which is independent of the first (i.e., not metastasis).

Stage Grouping for Non–Small Cell Lung Cancer

Once the T, N, and M categories have been assigned, this information is combined (stage grouping) to assign an overall stage of 0, I, II, III, or IV. The stages identify tumor types that have a similar prognosis and thus are treated in a similar way. Patients with lower stage numbers have a better prognosis.

Stage 0 - Tis, N0, M0

The cancer is found only in the layer of cells lining the air passages. It has not invaded other lung tissues or spread to lymph nodes or distant sites.

Stage IA - T1, N0, M0

The cancer is no larger than 3 cm, has not spread to the membranes that surround the lungs, does not affect the main branches of the bronchi, and has not spread to lymph nodes or distant sites.

Stage IB - T2, N0, M0

The cancer is larger than 3 cm, or involves a main bronchus but is not near the carina, or it has spread to the pleura, or the cancer is partially clogging the airways. It has not spread to lymph nodes or distant sites.

Stage IIA - T1, N1, M0

The cancer is no larger than 3 cm, has not spread to the membranes that surround the lungs, and does not affect the main branches of the bronchi. It has spread to nearby or hilar lymph nodes, but not to distant sites.

Stage IIB - T2, N1, M0 or T3, N0, M0

The cancer is larger than 3 cm or involves a main bronchus but is not near the carina, or it has spread to the pleura, or is partially clogging the airways. It has spread to nearby or hilar lymph nodes but not to distant sites; or it has spread to the chest wall or the diaphragm, the mediastinal pleura, or membranes surrounding the heart; or it invades a main bronchus and is close to the carina; or it has grown into the airways enough to cause an entire lung to collapse or to cause pneumonia in the entire lung. It has not spread to lymph nodes or distant sites.

Stage IIIA - T1 or 2, N2, M0 or T3, N1 or 2, M0

The cancer can be any size. It involves a main bronchus but is not near the carina, or it has spread to the pleura or is partially clogging the airways. It has spread to nodes in the middle of the chest (mediastinum) but not to distant sites; or it has spread to the chest wall or the diaphragm, the mediastinal pleura, or membranes surrounding the heart; or it invades a main bronchus and is close to the carina; or it has grown into the airways enough to cause an entire lung to collapse or to cause pneumonia in the entire lung. It has spread to lymph nodes anywhere in the chest on the same side as the cancer, but not to distant sites.

Stage IIIB - T1, 2 or 3, N3, M0 or T4, any N, M0

The cancer can be any size. It has spread to lymph nodes around the collarbone on either side or to hilar or mediastinal lymph nodes on the side opposite the cancerous lung; or it has spread to the mediastinum, the heart, the trachea, the esophagus, the backbone, or the carina; or two or more separate tumor nodules are present in the same lobe; or there is a fluid containing cancer cells in the space surrounding the lung. The cancer may or may not have spread to lymph nodes. It has not spread to distant sites.

Stage IV - Any T, Any N, M1

The cancer has spread to distant sites.

Non–Small Cell Lung Cancer Survival by Clinical Stage Based on Patients Diagnosed in 1992–1993

(These numbers come from the American College of Surgeons, National Cancer Data Base, published in the AJCC Manual, 6th edition.)

Stage	Relative 5-year Survival Rate
I	47%
II	26%
III	8%
IV	2%

The **5-year survival rate** refers to the percentage of patients who live at least 5 years after their cancer is diagnosed. Many patients live much longer than 5 years after diagnosis, and 5-year rates are used to produce a standard way of discussing prognosis. The **relative 5-year survival rate** assumes that people will die of other causes and compares the observed survival with that expected for people without lung cancer. That means that relative survival only talks about deaths from lung cancer. Of course, 5-year survival rates are based on patients diagnosed and initially treated more than 5 years ago. Improvements in treatment often result in a more favorable outlook for recently diagnosed patients.

Five-year survival rates will be higher for the A groups and lower for the B subgroups. It is also important to realize that the stage you are given is called a clinical stage. If you have surgery, the surgeon may find cancer in unsuspected areas. This would change your stage. This second and more accurate stage is called the pathologic stage.

Treatment

Your Medical Team

Your health care team will be made up of several people, each with different expertise to contribute to your care. One of your **cancer care team** members will take the lead in coordinating your care. Most lung cancer patients initially choose a medical oncologist to lead the team. It should be clear to all team members who is in charge, and that person should inform the others of your progress. This alphabetical list will acquaint you with the health care professionals you may encounter, depending on which treatment option and follow-up path you choose, and their areas of expertise:

Anesthesiologist

An anesthesiologist is a medical doctor who administers anesthesia (drugs or gases) to make you sleep and be unconscious or to prevent or relieve pain during and after a surgical procedure.

Dietitian

A dietitian is specially trained to help you make healthy diet choices and maintain a healthy weight before, during, and after treatment. A registered dietitian (RD) has at least a bachelor's degree and has passed a national competency exam.

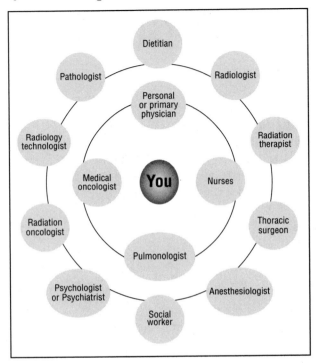

Medical Oncologist

A medical oncologist (also sometimes simply called an oncologist) is a medical doctor you may see after diagnosis. The oncologist is a cancer expert who understands specific types of cancer, their treatments, and their causes. He or she may help people with cancer make decisions about a course of treatment and then manage all phases of cancer care. Oncologists most often become involved when you need chemotherapy, but can also prescribe hormonal therapy and other anticancer drugs.

Nurses

During your treatment you will be in contact with different types of nurses.

Registered nurse

A registered nurse has an associate or bachelor's degree in nursing and has passed a state licensing exam. She or he can monitor your condition, provide treatment, educate you about side effects, and help you adjust to lung cancer physically and emotionally.

Nurse practitioner

A nurse practitioner is a registered nurse with a master's or doctoral degree who can manage lung cancer care and has additional training in primary care. He or she shares many tasks with your doctors, such as recording your medical history, conducting physical exams, and doing follow-up care. In most states, a nurse practitioner can prescribe medicines with a doctor's supervision.

Clinical nurse specialist

A clinical nurse specialist (CNS) is a nurse who has a master's degree in a specific area, such as oncology, psychiatry, or critical care nursing. The CNS often provides expertise to staff and may provide special services to patients, such as leading support groups and coordinating cancer care.

Oncology-certified nurse

An oncology-certified nurse is a clinical nurse who has demonstrated an in-depth knowledge of oncology care. He or she has passed a certification exam. Oncology-certified nurses are found in all areas of cancer practice.

Pathologist

A pathologist is a medical doctor specially trained in diagnosing disease based on the examination of microscopic tissue and fluid samples. He or she will determine the classification (cell type) of your cancer, help determine the stage (extent) and grade (estimate of aggressiveness) of your cancer, and issue a pathology report so that you and your doctor can decide on treatment options.

Personal or Primary Care Physician

A personal physician may be a general doctor, internist, or family practice doctor. He or she is often the medical doctor you first saw when you noticed symptoms of illness. This general or family practice doctor may be a member of your medical team, but a specialist is most often a patient's cancer care team leader.

Psychologist or Psychiatrist

A psychologist is a licensed mental health professional who is often part of the medical team. He or she provides counseling on emotional and psychological issues. A psychologist may have specialized training and experience treating people with cancer.

A psychiatrist is a medical doctor specializing in mental health and behavioral disorders. Psychiatrists provide counseling and can also prescribe medications.

Pulmonologist

A pulmonologist is a doctor who specializes in the diagnosis and treatment of lung diseases. A pulmonologist may have first diagnosed your lung cancer, and you may continue to see this doctor if you have breathing trouble related to the cancer or other lung problems.

Radiation Oncologist

A radiation oncologist is a medical doctor who specializes in treating cancer by using therapeutic radiation (high-energy x-rays or seeds). If you choose radiation, this member of your medical team evaluates you frequently during the course of treatment and at intervals afterward. The radiation oncologist will usually work closely with your oncologist. He or she helps you make decisions about radiation therapy options. A radiation oncologist is assisted by a radiation therapist during treatment and works with a radiation physicist, an expert who is trained in ensuring that the right dose of radiation treatment is delivered to you. The physicist is also assisted by a dosimetrist, a technician who helps plan and calculate the dosage, number, and length of your radiation treatments.

Radiation Therapist

A radiation therapist is a specially trained technician who works with the equipment that delivers radiation therapy. He or she positions your body during the treatment and administers the radiation therapy.

Radiologist

A radiologist is a medical doctor specializing in the use of imaging procedures (for example, diagnostic x-rays, ultrasound, magnetic resonance images, bone scans, and others) that produce pictures of internal body structures. He or she has special training in diagnosing cancer and other diseases and interpreting the results of imaging procedures. Your radiologist issues a radiology report describing the findings to your pulmonologist, medical oncologist, or radiation oncologist. The radiology images and report may be used to aid in diagnosis; to help classify and determine the extent of your lung cancer; to help locate tumors during procedures, surgery, and radiation treatment; or to look for the possible spread or recurrence of the cancer after treatment.

Radiology Technologist

A radiology technologist is a trained health care professional who assists the radiologist by positioning your body for x-rays and other procedures and developing and checking the images for quality. The radiologist then reads these images.

Social Worker

A social worker is a health specialist, usually with a master's degree, who is licensed or certified by the state in which he or she works. A social worker is an expert in coordinating and providing social services. He or she is trained to help you and your family deal with a range of emotional and practical challenges, such as finances, child care, emotional issues, family concerns and relationships, transportation, and problems with the health care system. If your social worker is trained in cancer-related problems, he or she can counsel you about your fears or concerns, help answer questions about diagnosis and treatment, and lead cancer support groups. You may communicate with your social worker during a hospital stay or on an outpatient basis.

Thoracic Surgeon

A thoracic surgeon is a doctor who specializes in performing chest surgery. This doctor will most likely do any tumor biopsies that are part of a lung cancer diagnosis. This doctor will also perform any surgical procedure necessary to remove cancerous lung tissue and lymph nodes (see section on Surgery, page 55).

How Is Non–Small Cell Lung Cancer Treated?

This information represents the views of the doctors and nurses serving on the American Cancer Society's Cancer Information Database Editorial Board. These views are based on their interpretation of studies published in medical journals, as well as their own professional experience.

The treatment information in this document is not official policy of the Society and is not intended as medical advice to replace the expertise and judgment of your cancer care team. It is intended to help you and your family make informed decisions, together with your doctor.

Your doctor may have reasons for suggesting a treatment plan different from these general treatment options. Don't hesitate to ask him or her questions about your treatment options.

If you have lung cancer, your treatment options (choices) are surgery, radiation therapy, chemotherapy, and targeted therapy, either alone or in combination, depending on the stage of your cancer.

After the cancer is found and staged, your cancer care team will discuss your treatment options with you. It is important to take time and think about all of your possible choices. In choosing a treatment plan, the most significant factor is the stage of the cancer. For this reason, it is very important that your doctor order all the tests needed to determine the cancer's stage. Other factors to consider include your overall physical health, **performance status**, likely **side effects** of the treatment, and the probability of curing the disease, extending life, or relieving symptoms. One thing to remember is that age alone should not be a barrier to treatment. Older people can benefit from treatment as much as younger people as long as their general health is good.

In considering your treatment options it is often a good idea to seek a second opinion. A second opinion may provide more information and help you feel more confident about the treatment plan you have chosen. Your doctor should not mind your doing this. In fact, some insurance companies require you to get a second opinion. If your first doctor has done tests, the results can be sent to the second doctor so that you will not have to have them done again. If you are in an HMO (health maintenance organization), find out about its policy concerning second opinions.

Surgery

Depending on the type and stage of a lung cancer, surgery may be used to remove the cancer along with some surrounding lung tissue and lymph nodes. Surgery is the only reliable method to cure NSCLC.

- If a section (lobe) of the lung is removed, the operation is called a **lobectomy**.
- If the entire lung is removed, the surgery is called a **pneumonectomy**.
- Removing part of a lobe is known as a **segmentectomy** or wedge **resection**.

Lymph nodes are also removed to look for spread of the cancer.

These operations require general anesthesia (you are "asleep") and a surgical incision is made in the chest (called thoracotomy). You will generally spend 1 to 2 weeks in the hospital. Possible complications include excessive bleeding, wound infections, and pneumonia. Because the surgeon must spread ribs to get to the lung, the incision will hurt for some time after surgery. Your activity will be limited for at least a month or two.

If your lungs are in good condition (other than the presence of the cancer) you can usually return to normal activities after a lobe or even an entire lung has been removed. However, if your lungs have been damaged and you have noncancerous diseases such as emphysema or chronic bronchitis (which are common among heavy smokers), you may become short of breath with activities. Pulmonary function tests are done before surgery to determine whether you will have enough healthy lung tissue remaining after surgery.

If you can't undergo a thoracotomy because of lung disease or other serious medical problems, or if the cancer is widespread, other types of surgery can be used to relieve some symptoms. For example, laser surgery can be used to relieve blockage of airways that may be causing pneumonia or shortness of breath.

If the lung cancer has spread to your brain and there is only one tumor, you may benefit from removal of the brain metastasis. This is done by surgery through a hole in the skull (craniotomy). It should only be done if the tumor can be removed without damage to vital areas of the brain that control movement, sensation, and speech, and only if the lung tumor can also be completely removed.

Recently, a less invasive procedure for treating early stage lung cancer has been developed. This is called video-assisted thoracic surgery. A small hollow tube with a video camera attached to the end can be placed through a small hole in the chest to help the surgeon see the tumor. Only small incisions are needed, so there is a little less pain after the surgery. Most experts recommend that only tumors smaller than 3 to 4 cm (about 1½ inches) be treated this way. The cure rate after this surgery seems to be the same as with older techniques. It is important, though, that the surgeon performing this procedure be experienced since it requires more technical skill than the standard surgery. An advantage of this surgery is a shorter hospital stay, usually around 5 days.

Sometimes fluid accumulates in the chest cavity and interferes with breathing. In order to remove the fluid and keep it from coming back, doctors will perform a procedure called **pleurodesis**. A small tube is placed in the chest, all the fluid removed, and either talc or a drug such as tetracycline or a chemotherapy drug is instilled into the chest cavity. These cause irritation and scarring that will seal the space and prevent fluid buildup. The tube is generally left in a day or two to drain any new fluid that might accumulate.

Radiation Therapy

Radiation therapy uses high-energy rays (such as x-rays) to kill cancer cells.

External beam radiation therapy uses radiation delivered from outside the body that is focused on the cancer. This is the type of radiation therapy most often used to treat a primary lung cancer or its metastases to other organs.

Brachytherapy uses a small pellet of radioactive material placed directly into the cancer or into the airway next to the cancer. This is usually done through a bronchoscope.

External beam radiation therapy is sometimes used as the main (primary) treatment of lung cancer, especially if your general health is too poor to undergo surgery. Brachytherapy can also be used to help relieve blockage of large airways by cancer.

After surgery, radiation therapy can be used to kill very small deposits of cancer that cannot be seen and removed during surgery. Radiation therapy can also be used to relieve (palliate) symptoms of lung cancer such as pain, bleeding, difficulty swallowing, cough, and problems caused by brain metastases. It is usually given in small daily doses over several weeks.

Side effects of radiation therapy might include mild skin problems, nausea, vomiting, and **fatigue**. Often these go away after a short while. Radiation might also make the side effects of chemotherapy worse. Chest radiation therapy may damage your lungs and cause difficulty breathing and shortness of breath. Your esophagus, which is located in the middle of your chest, will be exposed to radiation. For this reason, you might have difficulty swallowing during the treatment. This will improve after treatment is over.

Radiation therapy to large areas of the brain can sometimes change your brain function. You may notice memory loss, headache, difficulty thinking, or diminished sexual desire. Usually these symptoms are minor compared to those caused by a brain tumor; nevertheless, they can reduce your quality of life. Side effects of radiation therapy to the brain usually become most serious 1 or 2 years after treatment.

A special kind of radiation therapy called the "gamma knife" can be used instead of surgery for single brain metastases. In this procedure, multiple beams of radiation are focused on the tumor over a few minutes to hours. The head is kept in the same position by placing it in a rigid frame.

Chemotherapy

Chemotherapy is treatment with anticancer drugs given into a vein or by mouth. These drugs enter the bloodstream and go throughout the body, making this treatment useful for cancer that has spread or metastasized to organs beyond the lung. Depending on the type and stage of lung cancer, chemotherapy may be given as the main (primary) treatment or as an addition (adjuvant) to surgery.

Chemotherapy for lung cancer generally uses a combination of drugs. Doctors who prescribe these drugs (medical oncologists) generally use a combination of medicines that have proven to be more effective than a single drug. Doctors give chemotherapy in cycles, with each period of treatment followed by a recovery period. Chemotherapy cycles generally last about 21 to 28 days, and initial treatment typically involves 4 to 6 cycles. Chemotherapy is not recommended for patients in poor health (performance status 3–4). Advanced age is not a barrier, as long as the patient is not in poor health.

The drug combinations most frequently used for initial chemotherapy or targeted therapy for NSCLC are cisplatin or carboplatin combined with one of the following:

- Paclitaxel
- Docetaxel
- Gemcitabine
- Vinorelbine
- Irinotecan
- Etoposide
- Vinblastine
- Bevacizumab

In patients who cannot tolerate combination chemotherapy, single agent chemotherapy can be used.

Chemotherapy or targeted therapy used for second-line treatment (medicines used if the cancer continues to grow during or after initial chemotherapy) for NSCLC include the following drugs:

- Docetaxel alone
- Erlotinib
- Pemetrexed

Recent studies have shown that 2 drugs are as good as 3 and that using combinations with less severe side effects, such as gemcitabine with vinorelbine or paclitaxel, may be as effective for many patients as combinations containing cisplatin or carboplatin. Again, advanced age is no barrier to receiving these drugs as long as the person is in good general health.

Chemotherapy drugs kill cancer cells but also damage some normal cells. Therefore, your doctors will pay careful attention to avoiding or minimizing side effects. These depend on the type of drugs, the amount taken, and the length of treatment.

Temporary side effects might include nausea and vomiting, loss of appetite, loss of hair, and mouth sores. Some drugs cause severe diarrhea.

Because chemotherapy can damage the blood-producing cells of the bone marrow, you may have low blood cell counts. Low blood cell counts can increase your risk for the following:

- infection (due to a shortage of white blood cells)
- bleeding or bruising after minor cuts or injuries (due to a shortage of blood platelets)
- fatigue or shortness of breath (due to low red blood cell counts)

Since cisplatin, vinorelbine, docetaxel, or paclitaxel can damage nerves, you might feel numbness or tingling, particularly in your fingers and toes, and sometimes your arms and legs might feel weak (this is called peripheral neuropathy). You should report this, as well as any other side effects or changes you experience while getting chemotherapy, to your medical team.

Some side effects disappear within a few days after treatment. There are remedies for many of these temporary side effects of chemotherapy. For example, your doctor can prescribe drugs for you to prevent or lessen nausea and vomiting.

Targeted Therapy

In the past few years, much lung cancer research has been focused on drugs that are specifically targeted at cancer cells and interfere with their ability to grow. For example, erlotinib (Tarceva®)

has been recently approved by the Food and Drug Administration (FDA) for use in patients with NSCLC who are no longer responding to chemotherapy (this is usually determined after 1 or 2 different chemotherapy combinations). This drug is taken by mouth. Common side effects of erlotinib include skin rash and diarrhea.

Antiangiogenesis drugs

For cancers to grow, they must form new blood vessels to keep them nourished. There has been an intense search for drugs that block this new vessel growth. One such drug, bevacizumab (Avastin®), has recently been found to prolong survival of patients with advanced lung cancer when it is added to the standard chemotherapy **regimen**. But the drug causes bleeding, which means it cannot be used in patients who are coughing up blood, whose cancer has spread to the brain, or who are on "blood thinners" (anticoagulation therapy). It also cannot be used in patients with squamous cell cancer, because it leads to bleeding from this type of lung cancer.

Clinical Trials

The purpose of clinical trials

Studies of promising new or experimental treatments in patients are known as clinical trials. A clinical trial is only done when there is some reason to believe that the treatment being studied may be valuable to the patient. Treatments used in clinical trials are often found to have real benefits.

Researchers conduct studies of new treatments to answer the following questions:

- Is the treatment helpful?
- How does this new type of treatment work?
- Does it work better than other treatments already available?
- What side effects does the treatment cause?
- Are the side effects greater or less than the **standard therapy**?
- Do the benefits outweigh the side effects?
- In which patients is the treatment most likely to be helpful?

Types of clinical trials

There are 3 phases of clinical trials in which a treatment is studied before it is eligible for approval by the FDA.

Phase I clinical trials

The purpose of a phase I study is to find the best way to give a new treatment and how much of it can be given safely. The cancer care team watches patients carefully for any harmful side effects. The treatment has been well tested in lab and animal studies, but the side effects in patients are not completely known. Doctors conducting the clinical trial start by giving very low doses of the drug to the first patients and increasing the dose for later groups of patients until side effects appear. Although doctors are hoping to help patients, the main purpose of a phase I study is to test the safety of the drug.

Phase II clinical trials

These studies are designed to see if the drug works. Patients are given the highest dose that doesn't cause severe side effects (determined from the phase I study) and closely observed for an effect on the cancer. The cancer care team also looks for side effects.

Phase III clinical trials

Phase III studies involve large numbers of patients—often several hundred. One group (the **control group**) receives the standard (most accepted) treatment. The other group receives the new treatment. All patients in phase III studies are closely watched. The study will be stopped if the side effects of the new treatment are too severe or if one group has had much better results than the others.

If you are in a clinical trial, you will have a team of experts taking care of you and monitoring your progress very carefully. The study is especially designed to pay close attention to you.

However, there are some risks. No one involved in the study knows in advance whether the treatment will work or exactly what side effects will occur. That is what the study is designed to find out. While most side effects disappear in time, some can be permanent or even life threatening. Keep in mind, though, that even standard treatments have side effects. Depending on many factors, you may decide to enroll in a clinical trial.

Deciding to enter a clinical trial

Enrollment in any clinical trial is completely up to you. Your doctors and nurses will explain the study to you in detail and will give you a form to read and sign indicating your desire to take part. This process is known as giving your **informed consent**. Even after signing the form and after the clinical trial begins, you are free to leave the study at any time, for any reason. Taking part in the study does not prevent you from getting other medical care you may need.

To find out more about clinical trials, ask your cancer care team. The following are among the questions you should ask:

- Is there a clinical trial for which I would be eligible?
- What is the purpose of the study?
- What kinds of tests and treatments does the study involve?
- What does this treatment do? Has it been used before?
- Will I know which treatment I receive?
- What is likely to happen in my case with, or without, this new treatment?
- What are my other choices and their advantages and disadvantages?
- How could the study affect my daily life?
- What side effects can I expect from the study? Can the side effects be controlled?
- Will I have to be hospitalized? If so, how often and for how long?

- Will the study cost me anything? Will any of the treatment be free?
- If I am harmed as a result of the research, what treatment would I be entitled to?
- What type of long-term follow-up care is part of the study?
- Has the treatment been used to treat other types of cancers?

The American Cancer Society offers a clinical trials matching service for patients, their family, and friends. You can access this service on our Web site at http://clinicaltrials.cancer.org or by calling 1-800-303-5691. Based on the information you provide about your cancer type, stage, and previous treatments, this service can compile a list of clinical trials that match your medical needs. In finding a center most convenient for you, the service can also take into account where you live and whether you are willing to travel.

You can also get a list of current clinical trials by calling the National Cancer Institute's Cancer Information Service toll free at 1-800-4-CANCER or by visiting the NCI clinical trials Web site at www.cancer.gov/clinicaltrials.

Complementary and Alternative Therapies

Complementary and alternative therapies are a diverse group of health care practices, systems, and products that are not part of usual medical treatment. They may include products such as vitamins, herbs, or **dietary supplements**, or procedures such as acupuncture, massage, and a host of other types of treatment. There is a great deal of interest today in complementary and alternative treatments for cancer. Many are now being studied to find out if they are truly helpful to people with cancer.

You may hear about different treatments from family, friends, and others, which may be offered as a way to treat your cancer or to help you feel better. Some of these treatments are harmless in certain situations, while others have been shown to cause harm. Most of them are of unproven benefit.

The American Cancer Society defines **complementary therapy** or methods as those that are used along with your regular medical care. If these treatments are carefully managed, they may add to your comfort and well-being. **Alternative therapy** or methods are defined as those that are used instead of your regular medical care. Some of them have been proven not to be useful or even to be harmful, but are still promoted as "cures." If you choose to use these alternatives, they may reduce your chance of fighting your cancer by delaying, replacing, or interfering with regular cancer treatment.

Treatment Choices by Stage for Non–Small Cell Lung Cancer

If you smoke, it is important that you stop. Studies have shown that patients who continue to smoke after the diagnosis of lung cancer have worse outcomes than those who stop.

Stage 0

Because stage 0 NSCLC is limited to the lining layer of air passages and has not invaded the nearby lung tissue, it is curable by surgery alone. No chemotherapy or radiation therapy is needed.

You can be treated by segmentectomy or wedge resection (surgical removal of defined segments or small wedges). Cancers in some locations (where the windpipe divides into the left and right main bronchi) are difficult to remove completely by surgery without also removing an entire lung.

Killing cancer cells by sensitizing them with an injected chemical and activating the chemical by shining a bright light directly on the cancer (endoscopic **photodynamic therapy**) is being tested in this situation and may be a useful alternative to surgery for stage 0 cancers. If you are truly stage 0, treatment will probably cure you.

Stage I

If you have stage I NSCLC your treatment will probably be only surgery. This can be removal of the tumor by taking out one lung lobe (lobectomy) or by taking out part of a lung by doing a segmentectomy or wedge resection. Recently, 2 groups of doctors have reported that giving chemotherapy after surgery (**adjuvant therapy**) to patients with stage IB NSCLC reduces the chance the cancer will come back and slightly improves the chance of survival.

Segmentectomy or wedge resection is recommended only for treating the smallest stage I cancers and for patients with other medical conditions that make removing the entire lobe dangerous. Most surgeons believe it is better to perform a lobectomy if the patient can tolerate it.

Chemotherapy and/or radiation therapy may be recommended if the pathologists report that there were cancer cells at the edge of the specimen. This means that some cancer may have been left behind. Another approach would be to repeat the operation to ensure that all the cancer has been removed.

If you have serious medical problems, you may receive only radiation therapy as your main treatment.

Stage II

If you have stage II NSCLC you will have the cancer in your lungs surgically removed by lobectomy or by some less extensive surgery such as a segmentectomy. A wedge resection might be done if you cannot withstand lobectomy. Sometimes removing the whole lung (pneumonectomy) is needed. Any lymph nodes with cancer in them are also removed. The type of lymph node involvement and whether cancer cells are found at the edges of the removed tissues are important factors when planning the next step of treatment. After surgery, chemotherapy and/or radiation therapy may be used to destroy cancer cells left behind after surgery, especially if cancer cells are present at the edge of the tissue removed by surgery. Even if the edges of the sample have no detectable cancer cells, some doctors may recommend additional chemotherapy and/or radiation therapy.

If you have serious medical problems, you may receive only radiation therapy as your main treatment.

Stage IIIA

If you have stage IIIA NSCLC your treatment will depend on the size of the tumor, where the cancer is located in your lung, and which lymph nodes it has spread to. Surgery alone is not usually the chosen option if cancer is found in lymph nodes in the mediastinum during your work-up. Chemotherapy and radiation therapy are the standard of care. The role of surgery after chemotherapy with or without radiation therapy is still controversial but is being studied.

If positive lymph nodes in your mediastinum are discovered at the time of surgery, your surgeon may proceed with removal of the tumor and lymph nodes if he or she thinks all the cancer can be removed. Chemotherapy is usually given with or without radiation to all stage IIIA lung cancers, even if surgery cannot be done to remove the tumor(s).

Stage IIIB

Stage IIIB NSCLC has spread too widely to be completely removed by surgery. If you are in relatively good health you may be helped by combined chemotherapy and radiation therapy. In some cases, you may be able to have surgery to remove some, if not all, of the tumors after chemotherapy or radiation therapy is given. After surgery, chemotherapy and radiation (if not given before surgery) are recommended.

Chemotherapy is usually given with or without radiation to all stage IIIB lung cancers, even if surgery cannot be done to remove the tumors. Several clinical trials are in progress to determine the best treatment for people with this stage of lung cancer.

Stage IV

Because stage IV NSCLC has spread to distant organs, a cure is usually not possible. Treatment options depend on the site of the distant spread and the number of tumors. If any aggressive therapy is used, the goal of treatment should be clear to you and your family. If you are in otherwise good health, surgery, chemotherapy, and radiation therapy can help you live longer, even though these treatments won't cure you. In general, treatments will also help you to feel better by relieving symptoms.

If you have an airway blocked by cancer you can be treated by brachytherapy (radioactive seeds placed with a bronchoscope) or by using a laser passed through a bronchoscope to destroy the part of the cancer in your airway. External beam radiation therapy can also treat complications of cancer in the lungs as well as problems from metastatic growth such as bone pain and nervous system symptoms.

Patients in very poor health may have serious, life-threatening complications of chemotherapy. If you have extensive cancer or are in otherwise poor health, you might want to consider supportive or **palliative treatment**, perhaps through a **hospice** program. Many people with lung cancer are concerned about pain. As the cancer grows around certain nerves it may cause severe pain. However, you can effectively relieve this pain with medicine. Sometimes radiation therapy will help. It is important that you talk to your doctor and take advantage of these treatments.

If you have had chemotherapy and it is not working, you might also want to consider palliative care. A second kind of chemotherapy may help you feel better even if only for a brief time. Another option might be treatment with erlotinib (Tarceva®). This may be especially useful if you are a woman with adenocarcinoma and have never smoked.

Even if you have incurable lung cancer you should try to get the most out of your life by making every day count. That means you should be as free of symptoms as possible. If you want to continue anti-cancer treatment, you might think about taking part in a clinical trial of new chemotherapy drugs or other new treatments such as one that stops the formation of new blood vessels (**angiogenesis**); substances that interfere with growth factor action, or other related drugs; **immunotherapy**; or **gene therapy**. These are worthwhile options that may benefit you as well as future patients. Deciding on the right time to discontinue chemotherapy and focus on palliative care is never easy. Good communication with doctors, nurses, family, and clergy, as well as discussions with hospice staff, can help people facing this situation.

More Treatment Information

For more details on treatment options—including some that may not be addressed in this book—the National Comprehensive Cancer Network (NCCN) and the National Cancer Institute (NCI) are good sources of information.

The NCCN, made up of experts from 20 of the nation's leading cancer centers, develops cancer treatment guidelines for doctors to use when treating patients. These are available on the NCCN Web site (www.nccn.org).

The American Cancer Society collaborates with the NCCN to produce a version of some of these treatment guidelines, written specifically for patients and their families. These less-technical versions are available on both the NCCN Web site (www.nccn.org) and the ACS Web site (www.cancer.org). A print version can also be requested from the ACS at 1-800-ACS-2345.

The NCI provides treatment guidelines via its telephone information center (1-800-4-CANCER) and its Web site (www.cancer.gov). Detailed guidelines intended for use by cancer care professionals are also available on www.cancer.gov.

Questions To Ask

What Should You Ask Your Doctor About Non–Small Cell Lung Cancer?

It is important for you to have honest, open discussions with your cancer care team. They want to answer all of your questions, no matter how trivial you might think they are:

- ❏ What kind of lung cancer do I have?
- ❏ Has my cancer spread beyond the primary site?
- ❏ What is the stage of my cancer and what does that mean in my case?
- ❏ What treatment choices do I have?
- ❏ What do you recommend and why?
- ❏ What is my expected survival rate, based on my cancer as you view it?
- ❏ What risks or side effects are there to the treatments you suggest?
- ❏ What are the chances of recurrence of my cancer with these treatment plans?
- ❏ What should I do to be ready for treatment?

In addition to these sample questions, be sure to write down some of your own. For instance, you might want more information about recovery times so you can plan your work schedule. Or, you may want to ask about second opinions or about clinical trials for which you may qualify.

After Treatment

What Happens After Treatment for Non–Small Cell Lung Cancer?

Completing treatment can be both stressful and exciting. You will be relieved to finish treatment, yet it is hard not to worry about cancer coming back. This is a very common concern among those who have had cancer.

It may take a while before your confidence in your own recovery begins to feel real and your fears are somewhat relieved. You can learn more about what to look for and how to learn to live with the possibility of cancer coming back in the American Cancer Society document *Living with Uncertainty: The Fear of Cancer Recurrence*, available at 1-800-ACS-2345.

Follow-up Care

After your treatment is over, it is very important to keep all follow-up appointments. During these visits, your doctors will ask about symptoms, do physical exams, and order blood tests or imaging tests such as CT scans or x-rays. Follow-up is needed to check for cancer **recurrence** or spread, as well as possible side effects of certain treatments. This is the time for you to ask your health care team any questions you need answered and to discuss any concerns you might have.

Almost any cancer treatment can have side effects. Some may last for a few weeks to several months, but others can be permanent. Don't hesitate to tell your cancer care team about any symptoms or side effects that bother you so they can help you manage them.

It is also important to keep medical insurance. Even though no one wants to think of his or her cancer coming back, it is always a possibility. If it happens, the last thing you want is to have to worry about paying for treatment. Many people have been bankrupted by cancer recurrence. Should your cancer come back, the American Cancer Society document *When Your Cancer Comes Back: Cancer Recurrence* gives you information on how to manage and cope with this phase of your treatment. You can get this document by calling 1-800-ACS-2345.

Seeing a New Doctor

At some point after your cancer diagnosis and treatment, you may find yourself in the office of a new doctor. Your original doctor may have moved or retired, or you may have moved or changed doctors for some reason. It is important that you be able to give your new doctor the exact details of your diagnosis and treatment. Make sure you have the following information handy:

- a copy of your pathology report from any biopsy or surgery
- if you had surgery, a copy of your operative report
- if you were hospitalized, a copy of the discharge summary that every doctor must prepare when patients are sent home from the hospital
- finally, since some drugs can have long-term side effects, a list of your drugs, drug doses, and when you took them

After you show this to your new doctor, get your copies back and keep them in a safe place. You will likely need them again and again.

Lifestyle Changes to Consider During and After Treatment

Having cancer and dealing with treatment can be time-consuming and emotionally draining, but it can also be a time to look at your life in new ways. Maybe you are thinking about how to improve your health over the long term. Some people even begin this process during cancer treatment.

Make Healthier Choices

Think about your life before you learned you had cancer. Were there things you did that might have made you less healthy? Maybe you drank too much alcohol, or ate more than you needed, or smoked, or didn't exercise very often. Emotionally, maybe you kept your feelings bottled up, or maybe you let stressful situations go on too long.

Now is not the time to feel guilty or to blame yourself. However, you can start making changes *today* that can have positive effects for the rest of your life. Not only will you feel better but you will also be healthier. What better time than *now* to take advantage of the motivation you have as a result of going through a life-changing experience like having cancer?

You can start by working on those things that you feel most concerned about. Get help with those that are harder for you. For instance, if you are thinking about quitting smoking and need help, call the American Cancer Society's Quitline® tobacco cessation program at 1-800-ACS-2345.

Diet and Nutrition

Eating right can be a challenge for anyone, but it can get even tougher during and after cancer treatment. For instance, treatment often may change your sense of taste. Nausea can be a problem. You may lose your appetite for a while and lose weight when you don't want to. On the other hand, some people gain weight even without eating more. This can be frustrating too.

If you are losing weight or have taste problems during treatment, do the best you can with eating and remember that these problems usually improve over time. You may want to ask your cancer team for a referral to a dietitian, an expert in nutrition who can give you ideas on how to manage some of the side effects of your treatment. You may also find it helps to eat small portions every 2 to 3 hours until you feel better and can go back to a more normal schedule.

One of the best things you can do after treatment is to put healthy eating habits into place. You will be surprised at the long-term benefits of some simple changes, like increasing the variety of healthy foods you eat. Try to eat 5 or more servings of vegetables and fruits each day. Choose whole grain foods instead of white flour and sugars. Try to limit meats that are high in fat. Cut back on processed meats like hot dogs, bologna, and bacon. Get rid of them altogether if you can. If you drink alcohol, limit yourself to 1 or 2 drinks a day at the most. And don't forget to get some type of regular exercise. The combination of a good diet and regular exercise will help you maintain a healthy weight and keep you feeling more energetic.

Rest, Fatigue, Work, and Exercise

Fatigue is a very common symptom in people being treated for cancer. This is often not an ordinary type of tiredness but a "bone-weary" exhaustion that doesn't get better with rest. For some, this fatigue lasts a long time after treatment and can discourage them from physical activity.

However, exercise can actually help you reduce fatigue. Studies have shown that patients who follow an exercise program tailored to their personal needs feel physically and emotionally improved and can cope better.

If you are ill and need to be on bed rest during treatment, it is normal to expect your fitness, endurance, and muscle strength to decline some.

Physical therapy can help you maintain strength and range of motion in your muscles, which can help fight fatigue and the sense of depression that sometimes comes with feeling so tired.

Any program of physical activity should fit your own situation. An older person who has never exercised will not be able to take on the same amount of exercise as a 20-year-old who plays tennis 3 times a week. If you haven't exercised in a few years but can still get around, you may want to think about taking short walks.

Talk with your health care team before starting, and get their opinion about your exercise plans. Then, try to get an exercise buddy so that you're not doing it alone. Having family or friends involved when starting a new exercise program can give you that extra boost of support to keep you going when the push just isn't there.

If you are very tired, though, you will need to balance activity with rest. It is okay to rest when you need to. It is really hard for some people to allow themselves to do that when they are used to working all day or taking care of a household. (For more information about fatigue, please see the publication *Cancer-Related Fatigue and Anemia Treatment Guidelines for Patients.*

Exercise can improve both your physical and emotional health:

- It improves your cardiovascular (heart and circulation) fitness.
- It strengthens your muscles.
- It reduces fatigue.

- It lowers anxiety and depression.
- It makes you feel generally happier.
- It helps you feel better about yourself.

And long term, we know that exercise plays a role in preventing some cancers. The American Cancer Society, in its guidelines on physical activity for cancer **prevention**, recommends that adults take part in at least 1 physical activity for 30 minutes or more on 5 days or more of the week. Children and teens are encouraged to try for at least 60 minutes a day of energetic physical activity at least 5 days a week.

How About Your Emotional Health?

Once your treatment ends, you may find yourself overwhelmed by emotions. This happens to a lot of people. You may have been going through so much during treatment that you could only focus on getting through your treatment.

Now you may find that you think about the potential of your own death, or the effect of your cancer on your family, friends, and career. You may also begin to re-evaluate your relationship with your spouse or partner. Unexpected issues may also cause concern—for instance, as you become healthier and have fewer doctor visits, you will see your health care team less often. That can be a source of anxiety for some.

This is an ideal time to seek out emotional and social support. You need people you can turn to for strength and comfort. Support can come in many forms: family, friends, cancer support groups, church or spiritual groups, online support communities, or individual counselors.

Almost everyone who has been through cancer can benefit from getting some type of support. What's best for you depends on your situation and personality. Some people feel safe in peer-support groups or education groups. Others would rather talk in an informal setting, such as church. Others may feel more at ease talking one-on-one with a trusted friend or counselor. Whatever your source of strength or comfort, make sure you have a place to go with your concerns.

The cancer journey can feel very lonely. It is not necessary or realistic to go it all by yourself. And your friends and family may feel shut out if you decide not to include them. Let them in—and let in anyone else who you feel may help. If you aren't sure who can help, call your American Cancer Society at 1-800-ACS-2345, and we can put you in touch with an appropriate group or resource.

You can't change the fact that you have had cancer. What you can change is how you live the rest of your life—making healthy choices and feeling as well as possible, physically and emotionally.

What Happens if Treatment Is No Longer Working?

If cancer continues to grow after one kind of treatment, or if it returns, it is often possible to try another treatment plan that might still cure the cancer, or at least shrink the tumors enough to help you live longer and feel better. On the other hand, when a person has received several different medical treatments and the cancer has not fully responded, over time the cancer tends to become resistant to all treatment. At this time, it's important to weigh the possible limited benefit of a new treatment against the possible downsides, including continued doctor visits and treatment side effects.

Everyone has his or her own way of looking at this. Some people may want to focus on remaining comfortable during their limited time left.

This is likely to be the most difficult time in your battle with cancer—when you have tried everything medically within reason and it's just not working anymore. Although your doctor may offer you new treatment, you need to consider that at some point, continuing treatment is not likely to improve your health or change your prognosis.

If you want to continue treatment to fight your cancer as long as you can, you still need to consider the odds of more treatment having any benefit. In many cases, your doctor can estimate the response rate for the treatment you are considering. Some people are tempted to try more chemotherapy or radiation, for example, even when their doctors say that the odds of benefit are less than 1%. In this situation, you need to think about and understand your reasons for choosing this plan.

No matter what you decide to do, it is important that you be as comfortable as possible. Make sure you are asking for and getting treatment for any symptoms you might have, such as pain. This type of treatment is called palliative treatment.

Palliative treatment helps relieve these symptoms, but is not expected to cure the disease; its main purpose is to improve your quality of life. Sometimes, the treatments you get to control your symptoms are similar to the treatments used to treat cancer. For example, radiation therapy might be given to help relieve bone pain from bone metastasis. Or chemotherapy might be given to help shrink a tumor and keep it from causing a bowel obstruction. But this is not the same as receiving treatment to try to cure the cancer.

At some point, you may benefit from hospice care. Most of the time, this can be given at home. Your cancer may be causing symptoms or problems that need attention, and hospice focuses on your comfort. You should know that receiving hospice care doesn't mean you can't have treatment for the problems caused by your cancer or other health conditions. It just means that the focus of your care is on living life as fully as possible and feeling as well as you can at this difficult stage of your cancer.

Remember that maintaining hope is also important. Your hope for a cure may not be as bright, but there is still hope for good times with family and friends—times that are filled with happiness and meaning. In a way, pausing at this time in your cancer treatment is an opportunity to refocus on the most important things in your life. This is the time to do some things you've always wanted to do and to stop doing the things you no longer want to do.

Latest Research

What's New in Non–Small Cell Lung Cancer Research and Treatment?

Progress in prevention, early **detection**, and treatment based on current research is expected to save many thousands of lives each year. Lung cancer research is currently being done in medical centers throughout the world.

Prevention

At this time, many researchers believe that prevention offers the greatest opportunity to fight lung cancer. Although decades have passed since the link between smoking and lung cancers was clearly identified, scientists estimate that smoking is still responsible for about 85%–90% of lung cancers. Research is continuing in these areas:

- ways to help people quit smoking through counseling, nicotine replacement, and other medications
- ways to convince young people to never start smoking

- identifying inherited differences in genes that may make some people exceptionally likely to get lung cancer if they smoke or are exposed to someone else's smoke

Although researchers are looking for ways to use vitamins or medicine to prevent lung cancer in people at high risk, these have so far not proved successful. For now most researchers think that simply following the American Cancer Society dietary recommendations (such as choosing most foods from plant sources and eating at least 5 servings of fruits and vegetables each day) may be the best strategy.

Earlier Diagnosis

Nearly 20 years ago, large studies were done to determine whether routine chest x-rays and sputum cytology testing could save lives. Most researchers concluded that these tests did not find lung cancers early enough to significantly lower the risk of death from lung cancer. However, some researchers disagree about the best way to interpret the studies' data and the debate continues.

A large clinical trial called the National Lung Screening Trial (NLST) is underway to test whether spiral CT scanning of people at high risk of lung cancer will save lives. Information from this study will be coming out in the next few years. (For more information about the NLST, ask the American Cancer Society or the National Cancer Institute.) Another approach uses new ways to more sensitively detect cancer cells in sputum samples.

Researchers have recently found several changes that often affect the DNA of lung cancer cells. Current studies are evaluating new diagnostic tests that specifically recognize these DNA changes to see if this approach is useful in finding lung cancers at an earlier stage.

Treatment

Chemotherapy

Many clinical trials in progress are comparing the effectiveness of newer combinations of chemotherapy drugs. These studies will also provide information about minimizing side effects, especially in patients who are older and have other health problems. Clinical trials continue to search for better ways to combine chemotherapy with radiation therapy.

Targeted therapies

Researchers are learning more about the molecules within lung cancer cells that control their growth and spread in order to develop new targeted therapies. Several of these treatments are already being tested in clinical trials to see if they can help people with advanced lung cancer live longer or relieve their symptoms. Much remains to be learned about ways to combine these new targeted therapies with chemotherapy and radiation therapy, and this question is being addressed in laboratory experiments and in clinical trials. Several clinical trials have already reported that some patients do not benefit from certain targeted therapies, whereas others have quite remarkable shrinkage of their tumors. Researchers are now working on lab tests to help predict which patients will benefit from which drugs.

Antiangiogenesis drugs

In order for cancers to grow, blood vessels must develop to nourish the cancer cells. This process is called angiogenesis. New drugs that inhibit angiogenesis are under investigation as lung cancer treatments. Some have already been successfully used for other cancer types. A new drug called bevacizumab has shown some benefit in clinical trials of patients with non–small cell lung cancer and is currently being tested in small cell lung cancer. Other new drugs are being developed that may also be useful in stopping lung cancer growth by preventing new blood vessels from forming. Several of these drugs are being tested in clinical trials, and trials of new, more potent, antiangiogenesis drugs are expected to begin soon.

Vaccines

Many studies that try to get the body's immune system to fight the cancer are in progress. One that has been successful in NSCLC used patients' tumor cells to vaccinate patients against their own tumors. Others are using lung cancer cells that have been grown in the laboratory. In general these will probably be most effective in patients with early stage cancer, perhaps after surgery.

Resources

Additional Resources

More Information from Your American Cancer Society

The following related information may also be helpful to you. These materials may be ordered from our toll-free number, 1-800-ACS-2345.

After Diagnosis: A Guide for Patients and Families (also available in Spanish)

Caring for the Patient with Cancer at Home (also available in Spanish)

Pain Control: A Guide for People With Cancer and Their Families (also available in Spanish)

Questions About Smoking, Tobacco, and Health (also available in Spanish)

Understanding Chemotherapy (also available in Spanish)

Understanding Radiation Therapy (also available in Spanish)

The following books are available from the American Cancer Society. Call us at 1-800-ACS-2345 to ask about costs or to place your order.

American Cancer Society Consumer Guide to Cancer Drugs, Second Edition

American Cancer Society's Complementary and Alternative Cancer Methods Handbook

American Cancer Society's Guide to Pain Control: Understanding and Managing Cancer Pain, Revised Edition

Because... Someone I Love Has Cancer: Kids' Activity Book

Cancer in the Family: Helping Children Cope with a Parent's Illness

Cancer: What Causes It, What Doesn't

Caregiving: A Step-By-Step Resource for Caring for the Person with Cancer at Home, Revised Edition

Coming to Terms with Cancer: A Glossary of Cancer-Related Terms

Couples Confronting Cancer: Keeping Your Relationship Strong

Eating Well, Staying Well: During and After Cancer

Informed Decisions: The Complete Book of Cancer Diagnosis, Treatment, and Recovery, Second Edition

Kicking Butts: Quit Smoking and Take Charge of Your Health

Lymphedema: Understanding and Managing Lymphedema After Cancer Treatment

Our Mom Has Cancer

When the Focus Is on Care: Palliative Care and Cancer

National Organizations and Web Sites*

In addition to the American Cancer Society, other sources of patient information and support include:

American Lung Association
Telephone: 1-800-586-4872 or 1-212-315-8700
Internet address: www.lungusa.org

It's Time to Focus on Lung Cancer
> Telephone: 1-877-646-LUNG (1-877-646-5864)
> Internet address: www.lungcancer.org

Lung Cancer Alliance
> Telephone: 1-800-298-2436 (United States only)
> or 1-202-463-2080
> Internet address: www.lungcanceralliance.org

National Cancer Institute
> Telephone: 1-800-4-CANCER (1-800-422-6237)
> or TTY 1-800-332-8615
> Internet address: www.cancer.gov

*Inclusion on this list does not imply endorsement by the American Cancer Society

The American Cancer Society is happy to address almost any cancer-related topic. If you have any more questions, please call us at 1-800-ACS-2345, any time, any day.

References

Alberg AJ, Brock MV, Samet JM. Epidemiology of lung cancer: Looking to the future. *J Clin Oncol.* 2005;23:3175-3185

American Cancer Society. *Cancer Facts and Figures 2007.* Atlanta, Ga: American Cancer Society; 2007.

American Joint Committee on Cancer. Lung. *AJCC Cancer Staging Manual.* 6th ed. New York: Springer. 167-177.

NCCN Clinical Practice Guidelines in Oncology. Non Small Cell Lung Cancer. Version 2, 2006. www.nccn.org. Accessed August 2006.

Posther KE, Harpole DH. The surgical management of lung cancer. *Cancer Investigation.* 2006;24:56-57

Ruckdeschel JC, Schwartz AG, Bepler G, et al. Cancer of the lung: NSCLC and SCLC. In: Abeloff MD, Armitage JO, Lichter AS, Niederhuber JE. Kastan MB, McKenna WG. *Clinical Oncology*. 3rd ed. Philadelphia, Pa. Elsevier:2004:1649-1743.

Schrump DS, Altorki NK, Henschke CL, Carter D, Turrisi AT, Gutierrez ME. Non–small cell lung cancer. In: DeVita VT, Heilman S, Rosenberg SA, eds. *Cancer: Principles and Practice of Oncology*. 7th ed. Philadelphia, Pa: Lippincott Williams & Wilkins. 2005: 753-809.

U.S. Preventive Services Task Force. Lung cancer screening. *Ann Intern Med*. 2004;140:738-739.

Vaporciyan AA, Kiesw M,, Stevens CW, Komaki R, Roth JA. Cancer of the lung. In: Kufe DW, Pollock RE, Weichselbaum RR, Bast RC, Gansler TS, Holland JF, Frei E. *Cancer Medicine 6*. Hamilton, Ont: BC Decker; 2003. 1385-1446.

Your Small Cell Lung Cancer

What Is Cancer?

Cancer* develops when **cells** in a part of the body begin to grow out of control. Although there are many kinds of cancer, they all start because of out-of-control growth of abnormal cells.

Normal body cells grow, divide, and die in an orderly fashion. During the early years of a person's life, normal cells divide more rapidly until the person becomes an adult. After that, cells in most parts of the body divide only to replace worn-out or dying cells and to repair injuries.

Because a **cancer cell** continues to grow and divide, it is different from a normal cell. Instead of dying, cancer cells outlive normal cells and continue to form new abnormal cells.

Cancer cells often travel to other parts of the body where they begin to grow and replace normal **tissue**. This process, called **metastasis**, occurs when the cancer cells get into the bloodstream or **lymphatic system** of our body. However, when cells from a cancer like breast cancer spread to another organ like the liver, the cancer is still called breast cancer, not liver cancer.

* Terms in **bold type** are further explained in the dictionary that begins on page 175.

Cancer cells develop because of damage to **DNA**. This substance is in every cell and directs all its activities. Most of the time when DNA becomes damaged the body is able to repair it. In cancer cells, the damaged DNA is not repaired. People can inherit damaged DNA, which accounts for inherited cancers. Many times though, a person's DNA becomes damaged by exposure to something in the environment, like smoking.

Cancer usually forms as a **tumor**. Some cancers, like leukemia, do not form tumors. Instead, these cancer cells involve the blood and blood-forming organs and circulate through other tissues where they grow.

Remember that not all tumors are cancerous. A **benign** (non-cancerous) **tumor** does not spread to other parts of the body (**metastasize**) and, with very rare exceptions, is not life-threatening.

Different types of cancer can behave very differently. For example, lung cancer and breast cancer are very different diseases. They grow at different rates and respond to different treatments. That is why people with cancer need treatment that is aimed at their particular kind of cancer.

Cancer is the second leading cause of death in the United States. Nearly half of all men and a little over one-third of all women in the United States will develop cancer during their lifetimes. Today, millions of people are living with cancer or have had cancer. The risk of developing most types of cancer can be reduced by changes in a person's lifestyle, for example, by quitting smoking and eating a better diet. The sooner a cancer is found and treatment begins, the better a patient's chances of living for many years.

What Is Small Cell Lung Cancer?

Note: This section is specifically for the small cell type of lung cancer. The treatment for each type of lung cancer (small cell vs. non–small cell) is very different. So the information for one type will not apply to the other type. If you are not sure which type of lung cancer you have, it is very important to ask your doctor so you can be sure the information you receive is correct.

The Lungs

Your lungs are 2 sponge-like organs found in your chest. Your right lung is divided into 3 sections, called lobes. Your left lung has 2 lobes. It is smaller because your heart takes up more room on that side of the body. When you breathe, air goes into your lung through the **trachea** (windpipe). The trachea divides into tubes called the **bronchi**, which divide into smaller branches called the **bronchioles**. At the end of the bronchioles are tiny air sacs known as **alveoli**. Many tiny blood vessels run through the alveoli, absorbing oxygen from the inhaled air into your bloodstream and releasing carbon dioxide. Taking in oxygen and getting rid of carbon dioxide are your lungs' main functions. A lining, called the **pleura**, surrounds the lungs. This slippery lining protects your lungs and helps them slide back and forth as they expand and contract during breathing.

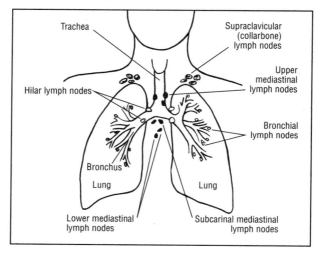

Most lung cancers start in the lining of the bronchi, but they can also begin in other areas such as the trachea, bronchioles, or alveoli. Lung cancers are thought to develop over a period of many years. First, there may be areas of **precancerous** changes in the lung. These changes do not form a mass or tumor. They cannot be seen on an **x-ray** and they do not cause **symptoms**. But these precancerous changes can be found by analyzing cells in the lining of the airways of smoke-damaged lungs.

Recently, molecular abnormalities believed to be precancerous have been identified in cells from people at **high risk** to develop lung cancers (for example, survivors from one prior lung cancer). These precancerous changes often progress to true cancer. As a cancer develops, the cancer cells may produce chemicals that cause new blood vessels to form nearby. These new blood vessels nourish the cancer cells, which can continue to grow and form a tumor large enough to be seen on x-rays. Cells from the cancer can break away from the original tumor and spread to other parts of the body. As noted earlier, this process is called metastasis. Lung cancer is a life-threatening disease because it often spreads in this way even before it can be detected on a chest x-ray.

One of the ways lung cancer can spread is through the lymphatic system. Lymphatic vessels are similar to veins but carry lymph instead of blood. Lymph is a clear fluid that contains tissue waste products and **immune system** cells. Lymphatic vessels of the lungs lead to nearby **lymph nodes** inside the chest. These nodes are located around the bronchi and in the **mediastinum** (the area between the 2 lungs). Cancer cells may enter lymph vessels and spread out along these vessels to reach lymph nodes. Lymph nodes are small, bean-shaped collections of immune system cells that are important in fighting infections. When lung cancer cells reach the lymph nodes, they can continue to grow. If cancer cells have multiplied in the lymph nodes, they are more likely to have spread to other organs of the body as well. **Staging** of the cancer and decisions about lung cancer treatment are based on whether the cancer has spread to the nearby lymph nodes in the mediastinum. These topics are discussed later in this book.

Types of Lung Cancer

There are 2 major types of lung cancer:

- small cell lung cancer (SCLC)
- non–small cell lung cancer (NSCLC)

If a lung cancer has characteristics of both types it is called a mixed small cell/large cell **carcinoma**. This is uncommon. These 2 main types of lung cancer are discussed separately because they are treated very differently.

Small Cell Lung Cancer

About 10%–15% of all lung cancers are the small cell type (SCLC), named for the small cells that make up these cancers. SCLC tends to spread widely through the body. This is important because it means that surgery is rarely an option (and never the only treatment given). Treatment must include drugs to kill the widespread disease. The cancer cells can multiply quickly, form large tumors, and spread to lymph nodes and other organs such as the bones, brain, adrenal glands, and liver. This type of cancer often starts in the bronchi near the center of the chest. Small cell lung cancer is almost always caused by smoking. It is very rare for someone who has never smoked to have small cell lung cancer. Other names for SCLC are oat cell carcinoma and small cell undifferentiated carcinoma.

Other Types of Lung Cancer

In addition to the 2 main types of lung cancer, other tumors can occur in the lungs. Some of these are non-cancerous (benign). **Carcinoid**

tumors of the lung account for fewer than 5% of lung tumors. Most are slow-growing tumors that are called typical carcinoid tumors. They are generally cured by surgery. Although some typical carcinoid tumors can spread, they usually have a better prognosis than small cell or non–small cell lung cancer. **Atypical** carcinoid tumors are much less common than typical carcinoids, but they are more likely to grow and spread quickly.

Cancer that has spread to the lungs from other organs (such as the breast, pancreas, kidney, or skin) is called **metastatic** cancer. Treatment for metastatic cancer to the lungs depends on where it started (the **primary site**).

What Are the Key Statistics About Lung Cancer?

During 2007, there will be about 213,380 new cases of lung cancer (both small cell and non–small cell), 114,760 among men and 98,620 among women. Lung cancer will account for about 15% of all new cancers. Lung cancer mainly occurs in the elderly. Nearly 70% of people diagnosed with lung cancer are older than 65; fewer than 3% of all cases are found in people under the age of 45. The average lifetime chance that a man will develop lung cancer is 1 in 12, and for a woman, it is 1 in 16. This figure includes all people and doesn't take into account whether or not they smoke.

Lung cancer is the leading cause of cancer death among both men and women. There will be an estimated 160,390 deaths from lung cancer

(89,510 among men and 70,880 among women) in 2007, accounting for around 29% of all cancer deaths. More people die of lung cancer than of colon, breast, and prostate cancers combined. Despite the very serious prognosis of lung cancer, some people are cured, and there are currently 330,000 long-term survivors.

Nearly 60% of people diagnosed with either type of lung cancer die within 1 year of their diagnosis. Nearly 75% die within 2 years. This has not improved in 10 years. Only about 6% of people diagnosed with small cell lung cancer survive this disease after 5 years.

Small cell lung cancer occurs slightly more often in men than women and equally in blacks and whites.

Risk Factors and Causes

What Are the Risk Factors for Small Cell Lung Cancer?

A **risk factor** is anything that increases your chance of getting a disease such as cancer. Different cancers have different risk factors. For example, unprotected exposure to strong sunlight is a risk factor for skin cancer. Several risk factors can make you more likely to develop lung cancer:

Tobacco Smoking

Smoking is by far the leading risk factor for lung cancer. At the beginning of the 20th century, lung cancer was a rare disease. The introduction of manufactured cigarettes, which made them readily available, changed this. About 87% of lung cancers are thought to result from smoking and some of the rest from passive exposure to tobacco smoke. The longer you smoke and the more packs per day you smoke, the greater your risk.

If you stop smoking before a cancer develops, your damaged lung tissue gradually starts to return to normal. Ten years after stopping smoking, your risk is reduced to one-third of what it would have been if you continued to smoke. Cigar smoking and pipe smoking are almost as likely to cause lung cancer as cigarette smoking. There is no evidence that smoking low tar cigarettes reduces the risk of lung cancer. There is concern that mentholated cigarettes may increase the risk. It is thought that the menthol may allow smokers to inhale more deeply.

If you don't smoke, but breathe in the smoke of others (called secondhand smoke or environmental tobacco smoke), you are also at increased risk for lung cancer. A nonsmoker who is married to a smoker has a 30% greater risk of developing lung cancer than the spouse of a nonsmoker. Workers who have been exposed to tobacco smoke in the workplace are also more likely to get lung cancer.

Hookah smoking has become popular among young people. It is actively marketed as safer than cigarettes because the percentage of tobacco in the product smoked is low and the smoke is filtered through water. However, experts at the American Cancer Society believe that smoking any amount of tobacco is dangerous. Studies have shown that hookah smoke contains the same cancer-causing substances as cigarettes. It is addictive and may lead to cigarette smoking in the future.

Asbestos

If you are an asbestos worker, you are about 7 times more likely to die of lung cancer. Exposure to asbestos fibers is an important risk factor for lung cancer. And if you are or have been an asbestos worker who smokes, your lung cancer risk is 50 to 90 times greater than that of people in general. Both smokers and nonsmokers exposed to asbestos also have a greater risk of developing a type of cancer that starts from the pleura (the layer of cells that line the outer surface of the lung). This cancer is called mesothelioma.

In recent years, government regulations have nearly stopped the use of asbestos in commercial and industrial products. It is still present in many homes and commercial buildings but is not considered harmful as long as it is not released into the air by deterioration, demolition, or renovation.

Arsenic
High levels of arsenic in drinking water may increase the risk of lung cancer. This effect is even more pronounced in smokers.

Radon
When uranium breaks down naturally it produces radon, a radioactive gas that cannot be seen, tasted, or smelled. Outdoors, there is so little radon that it is not dangerous. But indoors, radon can be more concentrated and become a possible risk for cancer. Recently, concerns have been raised about houses in some parts of the United States built over soil with natural uranium deposits that can create high indoor radon levels. Studies from these areas have found that the risk of lung cancer may double or even triple if you have lived for many years in a radon-contaminated house. This is a very small increase though, when it is compared to the lung cancer risk from tobacco.

Smokers are especially sensitive to the effects of radon. State and local offices of the Environmental Protection Agency can give you the names of reliable companies that perform radon testing and renovation.

Cancer-Causing Agents in the Workplace

Other **carcinogens** (cancer-causing agents) found in the workplace that can increase your lung cancer risk include the following:

- radioactive ores such as uranium
- inhaled chemicals or minerals such as beryllium, vinyl chloride, nickel chromates, coal products, mustard gas, and chloromethyl ethers
- fuels such as gasoline
- diesel exhaust

The government and industry have taken major steps in recent years to protect workers. But the dangers are still present, and if you work around these agents, you should be very careful to avoid exposure.

Marijuana

More tar is contained in marijuana than in cigarettes. Marijuana is also inhaled very deeply and the smoke is held in the lungs for a long time. Marijuana is smoked all the way to the end where tar content is the highest. Many of the cancer-causing substances in tobacco are also found in marijuana. Because marijuana is an illegal substance, it is not possible to control whether it contains pesticides and other additives. Medical reports suggest marijuana may cause cancers of the mouth and throat.

It has been hard to prove a connection between marijuana and lung cancer because it is not easy to gather information about the use of illegal drugs. Also, many marijuana smokers also smoke cigarettes. This makes it difficult to know how much of the risk is from tobacco and how much is from marijuana.

Radiation Therapy to the Lungs

People who have had **radiation therapy** to the chest for cancer are at higher risk for lung cancer, particularly if they smoke. Typical patients are those treated for **Hodgkin disease** or women who receive radiation to the chest after a mastectomy for breast cancer. Women who receive radiation therapy to the breast after a lumpectomy do not have a higher than expected risk of lung cancer. But if they smoke, their chance of lung cancer goes up markedly.

Talc and Talcum Powder

In the past, some studies suggested that talc miners and millers have a higher risk of lung cancer and other respiratory diseases because of their exposure to industrial grade talc. Recent studies of talc miners have not found an increase in lung cancer rate. Talcum powder is made from talc, a mineral that in its natural form may contain asbestos. By law since 1973, all home-use talcum products (baby, body, and facial powders) have been asbestos-free. The use of cosmetic talcum powder has not been found to increase your risk of lung cancer.

Other Mineral Exposures

People with silicosis and berylliosis (lung diseases caused by breathing in certain minerals) also have a higher risk of lung cancer.

Personal and Family History of Lung Cancer

If you have had lung cancer, you have a higher risk of developing another lung cancer. Brothers, sisters, and children of those who have had lung cancer may have a slightly higher risk of lung cancer themselves. Recently, a group called the Genetic Epidemiology of Lung Cancer Consortium studied families with a strong history of lung cancer. They found that the susceptibility to lung cancer might reside on a particular **chromosome** (chromosome 6). People who have this abnormality on chromosome 6 will more readily develop lung cancer even if they only smoke a little. Other family members who lack the genetic abnormality have to smoke more to develop lung cancer.

Another study, conducted in Iceland, found that if a person's **first degree relative** (sibling, parent) had lung cancer, that person's chance of developing the disease doubles. Other studies have shown that the risk of lung cancer increases in a family if someone in the family developed the cancer at a young age.

Diet

Some reports have indicated that a diet low in fruits and vegetables may increase the chances of getting cancer if you are exposed to tobacco smoke.

Evidence is growing that fruits and vegetables may protect you against lung cancer.

Air Pollution

In some cities, air pollution can slightly increase the risk of lung cancer. This risk is far less than that caused by smoking.

Do We Know What Causes Small Cell Lung Cancer?

Tobacco smoking is by far the leading cause of lung cancer. Almost all small cell lung cancers are caused directly by smoking. Other risk factors for lung cancer include a family history or personal history of lung cancer and exposure to cancer-causing agents in the workplace or the environment.

Recently, scientists have begun to understand how these risk factors produce certain changes in the DNA of cells in the lungs, causing them to grow abnormally and form cancers. DNA is the genetic material that carries the instructions for nearly everything our cells do. We usually resemble our parents because they passed their DNA on to us. However, DNA affects more than our outward appearance. Some genes (parts of our DNA) contain instructions for controlling when cells grow and divide.

Genes that promote cell division are called **oncogenes**. Genes that slow down cell division or cause cells to die at the appropriate time are called **tumor suppressor genes**.

Cancer can be caused by a DNA **mutation** (defect) that activates (turns on) oncogenes or inactivates (turns off) tumor suppressor genes. Some people inherit DNA mutations from their parents that greatly increase their risk for developing breast, ovarian, colorectal, and several other cancers. However, inherited oncogene or tumor suppressor gene mutations are not believed to cause very many lung cancers.

Oncogene and tumor suppressor gene mutations related to lung cancer usually develop during life rather than before birth as an inherited mutation. Every time a cell prepares to divide into 2 new cells, it must duplicate its DNA. This process is not perfect and copying errors occur.

Fortunately, cells have repair enzymes that proofread the DNA, but some errors may slip past. Some people may have faulty DNA repair mechanisms that make them especially vulnerable to cancer-causing chemicals and radiation. Acquired mutations in lung cells often result from exposure to cancer-causing chemicals in tobacco smoke. Acquired changes in genes, such as the *p53* tumor suppressor gene and the *ras* oncogene, are thought to be important in the development of lung cancer. Changes in these and similar genes may also make some lung cancers likely to grow and invade more rapidly than others.

Although inherited mutations of oncogenes or tumor suppressor genes rarely cause lung cancers, some people seem to inherit a reduced ability to detoxify (break down) certain types of cancer-causing chemicals.

Other people may inherit an increased tendency to activate carcinogens, making these genes even more dangerous. These people are more sensitive to the cancer-causing effects of tobacco smoke and certain industrial chemicals. Researchers are developing tests that may help identify such people, but these tests are not yet reliable enough for routine use. Therefore, doctors recommend that all people avoid tobacco smoke and hazardous industrial chemicals.

Prevention and Detection

Can Small Cell Lung Cancer Be Prevented?

The best way to prevent lung cancer is to not smoke and to avoid breathing in other people's smoke. If you already smoke, you should quit. Likewise, working and living in an environment free of cancer-causing chemicals will also be helpful. A healthy diet with lots of fruits and vegetables may also help prevent this cancer.

There have been many attempts to reduce the risk of lung cancer in current or former smokers by giving them high doses of vitamins or vitamin-like drugs. These have been completely unsuccessful. In one study, a nutrient related to vitamin A, called *beta-carotene*, appeared to increase the rate of cancer.

Some people who get lung cancer do not have any apparent risk factors. Although we know how to prevent most lung cancers, at this time we don't know how to prevent all of them.

Can Small Cell Lung Cancer Be Found Early?

Usually symptoms of lung cancer do not appear until the disease is in an **advanced stage**. But some lung cancers are diagnosed early because they are found as a result of tests for other medical conditions. For example, a diagnosis may be made by an **imaging test** or a **scan** (such as a chest x-ray or chest **CT scan**), **bronchoscopy** (viewing the inside of bronchi through a flexible lighted tube), or **sputum cytology** (microscopic examination of cells in coughed up phlegm) performed for other reasons in patients with heart disease, pneumonia, or other lung conditions.

Screening Tests for Lung Cancer

Screening is the use of tests or examinations to detect a disease in people without symptoms of that disease. For example, the Pap test is used to screen for cervical cancer. Because lung cancer usually spreads beyond the lungs before causing any symptoms, an effective screening program to detect lung cancer early could save many lives.

Thus far, no lung cancer screening test has been shown to prevent people from dying of this disease. The use of chest x-rays and sputum cytology (checking phlegm under the microscope to find cancer cells) has been tested for several years. The studies, which have been recently updated, have concluded that these tests could not find many lung cancers early enough to improve a person's chance for a cure. For this reason, lung cancer screening is not a routine practice for the general public or even for people at increased risk, such as smokers.

Recently, a new x-ray technique called spiral or helical low-dose CT scanning has been successful in detecting early lung cancer in smokers and former smokers. But it has not yet been shown whether this technique will lower the chances of dying from lung cancer. One major problem with this test is that it finds a lot of abnormalities that turn out to not be cancer. This leads to a lot of unnecessary testing and even surgery.

A large **clinical trial** called the National Lung Screening Trial (NLST) is testing whether spiral CT scanning of people at high risk of lung cancer will save lives. This trial, which began in 2002, has studied about 50,000 people. It is now closed to new subjects. Soon we will learn whether spiral CT scanning will catch lung cancer early enough to save lives. Until this information is available, people who are interested in testing should understand the limits and benefits of low-dose CT scanning.

The United States Preventive Services Task Force (USPSTF), a group of experts gathered together by the U.S. government, recently concluded that no one has shown that screening for lung cancer helps patients. Their statement:

"The USPSTF recommends neither for nor against using chest x-ray, computed tomography (CT scan), or sputum cytologic examination to look for lung cancer in people who have no symptoms to suggest the disease. If screening is being considered, doctors and patients should discuss the pros and cons of screening before going ahead with x-ray, CT scan, or sputum cytologic examination to screen for lung cancer. Patients should be aware that there are no studies showing that screening helps people live longer. They should also know that **false-positive** test results are common and can lead to unnecessary worry, testing, and surgery."

People who are current smokers also should realize that the best way to avoid dying of lung cancer is to stop smoking. This is the surest route to good health.

The American Cancer Society recommends that, as much as possible, people who were smokers, are current smokers, have been exposed to second-hand smoke, or have worked around materials that increase the risk for lung cancer, be aware of their continuing lung cancer risk. These individuals should talk with their doctors about their likelihood of developing lung cancer and about the potential benefits and risks of lung cancer screening. The most obvious potential benefit is detection of some lung cancers at an early stage. Some studies have shown that CT scans can find lung cancer when most cases are curable. The main risk is that many of the scans will produce inconclusive findings that will need to be resolved by further tests that are invasive, uncomfortable, expensive, and have side effects that can be serious and even fatal. After a discussion about what is and is not known about the value of testing for early lung cancer detection, if you and your doctor decide in favor of testing, then be sure to choose an institution that has experience in lung scanning and that supports a multidisciplinary program dedicated to evaluation of high-risk individuals.

Diagnosis and Staging

How Is Small Cell Lung Cancer Diagnosed?

If there is a reason to suspect you may have lung cancer, your doctor will use one or more methods to find out if the disease is really present. In addition, a **biopsy** of the lung tissue can confirm the **diagnosis** of cancer and also give valuable information that will help in making treatment decisions. If these tests find lung cancer, more tests will be done to find out how far the cancer has spread.

Common Signs and Symptoms of Lung Cancer

Although most lung cancers do not cause any symptoms until they have spread too far to be cured, symptoms do occur in some people with early lung cancer. If you go to your doctor when you first notice symptoms, your cancer might be diagnosed and treated while it is in a curable stage. Or, at the least, you could live longer with a better **quality of life**. These are the most common symptoms of lung cancer:

- a cough that does not go away
- chest pain, often aggravated by deep breathing, coughing, and even laughing
- hoarseness
- weight loss and loss of appetite
- bloody or rust-colored sputum (spit or phlegm)
- shortness of breath
- recurring infections such as bronchitis and pneumonia
- new onset of wheezing

When lung cancer spreads to distant organs, it may cause these effects:

- bone pain
- neurologic changes (such as headache, weakness or numbness of a limb, dizziness, or recent onset of a seizure)
- jaundice (yellow coloring of the skin and eyes)
- masses near the surface of the body, due to cancer spreading to the skin or to lymph nodes (collection of immune system cells) in the neck or above the collarbone

If you have any of these problems, see your doctor right away. These symptoms could be the first warning of a lung cancer. Many of these symptoms can also result from other causes or from noncancerous diseases of the lungs, heart, and other organs. Seeing a doctor is the only way to find out. Other symptoms are listed below.

Horner syndrome

Cancer of the upper part of the lungs may damage a nerve that passes from the upper chest into your neck. Doctors sometimes call these cancers Pancoast tumors. Their most common symptom is severe shoulder pain. Sometimes they also cause Horner syndrome. Horner syndrome is the medical name for the group of symptoms consisting of drooping or weakness of one eyelid, reduced or absent perspiration on the same side of your face, and a smaller pupil (dark part in the center of the eye) on that side.

Paraneoplastic syndromes

Some lung cancers may produce **hormone**-like or other substances that enter the bloodstream and cause problems with distant tissues and organs, even though the cancer has not spread to those tissues or organs. These problems are called paraneoplastic (Latin for "tumor-related") syndromes. Sometimes these syndromes may be the first symptoms of early lung cancer. Because the symptoms affect other organs, patients and their doctors may first suspect that diseases other than lung cancer are causing them.

Patients with small cell lung cancer and those with non–small cell lung cancer often have different paraneoplastic syndromes. These are the most common paraneoplastic syndromes associated with small cell lung cancer:

- SIADH (syndrome of inappropriate anti-diuretic hormone) causes salt levels of the blood to become very low. Symptoms of SIADH include fatigue, loss of appetite, muscle weakness or cramps, nausea, vomiting, restlessness, and confusion. Without treatment, severe cases may lead to seizures and coma. The cause of this condition is a hormone made by the cancer which causes the kidneys to retain water.

- Ectopic Cushing syndrome causes excess production of certain hormones by the adrenal gland. Symptoms include weight gain, weakness, and high blood pressure. It is caused when the cancer produces ACTH, the hormone that makes the adrenal gland secrete cortisol.

- Some people develop neurologic problems such as unexplained loss of balance and unsteadiness in arm and leg movement (cerebellar degeneration). Another possible problem is a muscle disorder called Lambert-Eaton syndrome. In this problem, muscles around the hips become weak. One of the first signs is trouble getting up from a sitting position. Later, muscles around the shoulder may become weak too.

Many of these problems will improve with successful treatment of the cancer.

Medical History and Physical Exam

Your doctor will take a medical history (health-related interview) to check for risk factors and symptoms. Your doctor will also examine you to look for signs of lung cancer and other health problems.

Imaging Tests

Imaging tests use x-rays, magnetic fields, or radioactive substances to create pictures of the inside of your body. Several imaging tests are used to find lung cancer and determine where it may have spread in the body.

Chest x-ray

This is the first test your doctor will order to look for any mass or spot on the lungs. It is a plain x-ray of your chest and can be done in any outpatient setting. If the x-ray is normal, you probably don't have lung cancer. If something suspicious is seen, your doctor may order additional tests.

Computed tomography

Computed tomography (CT) is an x-ray procedure that produces detailed cross-sectional images of your body. Instead of taking one picture, as does a conventional x-ray, a CT scanner takes many pictures as it rotates around you. A computer then combines these pictures into an image of a slice of your body. The machine will take pictures and form multiple images of the part of your body that is being studied. Often after the first set of pictures is taken, you will receive an **intravenous** injection of a "dye" or radiocontrast agent that helps better outline structures in your body. A second set of pictures is then taken.

CT scans take longer than regular x-rays and you will need to lie still on a table while they are being done. But just like other computerized devices, they are getting faster and your stay might be pleasantly short. The newest CT scans take only seconds to complete. Also, you might feel a bit confined by the ring-like equipment you're in when the pictures are being taken.

The contrast "dye" is injected through an IV line. Some people are allergic to the dye and get hives, a flushed feeling, or, rarely, more serious reactions like trouble breathing and low blood pressure. Be sure to tell your doctor if you have ever had a reaction to any contrast material used for x-rays. If you have, you may need medicine before you can have such an injection during your test.

You may also be asked to drink a contrast solution. This helps outline your intestine if your doctor is looking at organs in your abdomen to see if the lung cancer has spread.

The CT scan will provide precise information about the size, shape, and position of a tumor and can help find enlarged lymph nodes that might contain cancer that has spread from the lung. CT scans are more sensitive than a routine chest x-ray in finding early lung cancers. This test is also used to find masses in the adrenal glands, brain, and other internal organs that may be affected by the spread of lung cancer.

Magnetic resonance imaging

Magnetic resonance imaging (MRI) uses radio waves and strong magnets instead of x-rays. The energy from the radio waves is absorbed and then released in a pattern formed by the type of tissue and by certain diseases. A computer translates the pattern of radio waves given off by the tissues into a very detailed image of parts of the body. Not only does this produce cross-sectional slices of the body like a CT scanner, it can also produce slices that are parallel with the length of your body.

A contrast material might be injected just as with CT scans, but is used less often. MRI scans take longer—often up to an hour. Also, you have to be placed inside a tube-like piece of equipment, which is confining and can upset people with claustrophobia. The machine makes a thumping noise that you may find annoying. Some places will provide headphones with music to block this out. MRI images are particularly useful in detecting lung cancer that has spread to the brain or spinal cord.

Positron emission tomography

Positron emission tomography (PET) uses glucose (a form of sugar) that contains a radioactive atom. A small amount of the radioactive material is injected into a vein. Cancer cells in the body absorb large amounts of the radioactive sugar and a special camera can detect the radioactivity. This can be a very important test if you have early-stage lung cancer. Your doctor will use this test to see if the cancer has spread to lymph nodes. It is also helpful in telling whether a shadow on your chest x-ray is cancer. A **PET scan** is also useful when your doctor thinks the cancer has spread, but doesn't know where. PET scans can be used instead of several different x-rays because they scan your whole body. Newer devices combine a CT scan and a PET scan to better pinpoint the tumor.

Bone scans

In a bone scan, a small amount of radioactive substance (usually technetium diphosphonate) is injected into a vein. The amount of radioactivity used is very low and causes no long-term effects. This substance builds up in areas of bone that may be abnormal because of cancer metastasis. Areas of diseased bone will be seen on the bone scan image as dense, gray to black areas, called "hot spots." These areas may suggest the presence of metastatic cancer, but arthritis, infection, or other bone diseases can also cause a similar pattern. Bone scans are routinely done in patients with small cell lung cancer. Usually, they are only done in patients with non–small cell lung cancer when other test results or symptoms suggest that the cancer has spread to the bones.

Procedures That Sample Tissues and Cells

One or more of these tests will be used to confirm that a lung mass seen on imaging tests is, indeed, lung cancer. These tests collect cells from the suspicious area and are also used to determine the exact type of lung cancer you may have and how far it may have spread. A **pathologist**, a doctor who specializes in laboratory tests to diagnose diseases such as cancer, will examine the cells using a microscope. If you have any questions about your pathology results or any diagnostic tests, do not hesitate to ask your doctor. You can get a second opinion of your pathology report, called a pathology review, by having your tissue specimen sent to another laboratory recommended by your doctor.

Sputum cytology

A sample of phlegm (mucus you cough up from the lungs) is examined under a microscope to see if cancer cells are present. The best way to do this is to get early morning samples from you 3 days in a row.

Needle biopsy

A needle can be guided into the suspicious area while your lungs are being looked at with fluoroscopy (fluoroscopy is like an x-ray, but the image is shown on a screen rather than on film). CT scans can also be used to guide the placement of needles. Unlike fluoroscopy, CT doesn't provide a continuous picture, so the needle is inserted in the direction of the mass, a CT image is taken, and the direction of the needle is guided based on the image. This process is repeated a few times until the CT image confirms that the needle is within the mass. A tiny sample of the target area is sucked into a syringe and examined under the microscope to see if cancer cells are present.

A thin needle can also be inserted through the wall of the trachea to sample nearby lymph nodes using a flexible, lighted tube called a bronchoscope.

This procedure, called **transtracheal fine needle aspiration**, is often used to take samples of subcarinal lymph nodes (around the point where the windpipe branches into the left and right bronchi) and mediastinal lymph nodes (along the windpipe and the major bronchial tube areas). (See illustration, page 98.)

Bronchoscopy

You will need to be sedated for this exam. A bronchoscope is passed through your mouth into the bronchi (the larger tubes which carry air to the lungs). This can help find some tumors or blockages in the lungs. At the same time, it can also be used in performing a biopsy (taking samples of tissue) or taking samples of lung secretions to be examined under a microscope for cancer cells or precancerous cells. Studies are being done to see if annual exams will be helpful in finding **premalignant** changes in people at high risk.

Endobronchial ultrasound

In this bronchoscopy technique, the bronchoscope is fitted with an **ultrasound** emitter and receiver at its tip. This may be helpful in gauging the size of the tumor and in spotting enlarged lymph nodes. A fine needle passed through the biopsy channel can sample these nodes under ultrasound guidance. This is usually not done for small cell lung cancer.

Endoscopic esophageal ultrasound

In **endoscopic esophageal ultrasound (EUS)**, the bronchoscope is fitted with an ultrasound emitter and receiver at its tip and passed into the esophagus. This is done with light sedation. The esophagus is close to some lymph nodes inside the chest, and lung cancer can spread to these lymph nodes. Ultrasound images taken from inside the esophagus can be helpful in finding large lymph nodes inside the chest that might contain metastatic lung cancer. A fine needle passed through a channel on the scope can sample these nodes under ultrasound guidance.

Mediastinoscopy and mediastinotomy

For both of these procedures, you will receive general **anesthesia** (be put into a deep sleep). With **mediastinoscopy** a small cut is made in your neck and a hollow lighted tube is inserted behind the sternum (breastbone). Special instruments operated through this tube can be used to take a tissue sample from the mediastinal lymph nodes (along the windpipe and the major bronchial tube areas). Looking at the samples under a microscope can show whether cancer cells are present. This is usually not done for small cell lung cancer.

With **mediastinotomy**, the surgeon removes samples of mediastinal lymph nodes while the patient is under general anesthesia. Unlike mediastinoscopy, with mediastinotomy the surgeon opens the chest cavity by making a small incision beside the sternum. This allows the surgeon to reach lymph nodes that are not reached by standard mediastinoscopy. This is usually not done for small cell lung cancer.

Thoracentesis and thoracoscopy

Thoracentesis and **thoracoscopy** are done to find out whether a buildup of fluid around the lungs (pleural effusion) is the result of cancer spreading to the membranes that cover the lungs (pleura). The buildup might also be caused by a condition such as heart failure or an infection.

For thoracentesis, the skin is numbed and a needle is placed between the ribs to drain the fluid. The fluid is checked under a microscope to look for cancer cells.

Chemical tests of the fluid are also sometimes useful in distinguishing a **malignant** pleural effusion from a benign one. Once malignant (cancerous) pleural fluid has been diagnosed, thoracentesis may be repeated to remove more fluid. Fluid buildup can prevent the lungs from filling with air, so thoracentesis can help the patient breathe better.

Thoracoscopy is a procedure that uses a thin, lighted tube connected to a video camera and monitor to view the space between the lungs and the chest wall. Using this, the doctor can see cancer deposits and remove a small piece of the tissue to be examined under the microscope. Thoracoscopy can also be used to sample lymph nodes and fluid.

Bone marrow biopsy

A needle is used to remove a sample of bone about $\frac{1}{16}$ inch across and 1 inch long (usually from the back of your hip bone) after the area has been numbed with local anesthesia. The sample is checked under the microscope for cancer cells. This procedure is done mostly to help in finding spread of small cell lung cancer.

Blood counts and blood chemistry

A complete **blood count** (CBC) determines whether your blood has the correct number of various cell types. For example, it can show if you have anemia. This test will be repeated regularly if you are treated with **chemotherapy**, because these drugs temporarily affect blood-forming cells of the bone marrow. The blood chemistry tests can spot abnormalities in some of your organs. If cancer has spread to the liver and bones, it may cause certain chemical abnormalities in the blood. If one of these in particular, called the LDH, is elevated, it usually means that the outlook for cure or long-term survival isn't as good.

How Is Small Cell Lung Cancer Staged?

Staging is the process of finding out how localized or widespread your cancer is. It describes how far the cancer has spread. Your treatment and prognosis (the outlook for chances of survival) depend, to a large extent, on the cancer's stage. The tests just described are used to stage the cancer.

Staging of Small Cell Lung Cancer

Although most cancers are staged with a 4-stage system that describes the tumor size, lymph node spread, and distant spread, this usually isn't done for small cell lung cancer. Instead, most doctors prefer a 2-stage system. These are limited stage and extensive stage. Limited stage usually means that the cancer is only in one lung and in lymph nodes on the same side of the chest.

Spread of the cancer to the other lung, to lymph nodes on the other side of the chest, or to distant organs indicates extensive disease. Many doctors consider small cell lung cancer that has spread to the fluid around the lung an extensive stage.

Small cell lung cancer is staged in this way because it helps separate patients who have a fair prognosis, can be treated with radiation therapy in addition to chemotherapy, and may be cured, from those who have a worse outlook with very little chance of cure. About two-thirds of the people with small cell lung cancer have extensive disease when their cancer is first found.

Relative Survival Rates

If small cell lung cancer is found very early and is apparently localized to the lung alone without any spread to lymph nodes, the **relative 5-year survival rate** is around 21%. Only 6% of patients fall into this category. If small cell lung cancer has shown any signs of spread, the relative 5-year survival rate is around 11%. Thirty-four percent of patients are in this class. For patients with extensive disease, the relative 5-year survival rate is 2%. These descriptions are not completely reliable though. How extensive a patient's cancer is depends partly on how hard doctors look for spread.

The relative 5-year survival rate assumes that people will die of other causes and compares the observed survival with that expected for people without lung cancer. That means that relative survival only talks about deaths from lung cancer.

Treatment

Your Medical Team

Your health care team will be made up of several people, each with different expertise to contribute to your care. One of your **cancer care team** members will take the lead in coordinating your care. Most lung cancer patients initially choose a medical oncologist to lead the team. It should be clear to all team members who is in charge, and that person should inform the others of your progress. This alphabetical list will acquaint you with the health care professionals you may encounter, depending on which treatment option and follow-up path you choose, and their areas of expertise:

Anesthesiologist

An anesthesiologist is a medical doctor who administers anesthesia (drugs or gases) to make you sleep and be unconscious or to prevent or relieve pain during and after a surgical procedure.

Dietitian

A dietitian is specially trained to help you make healthy diet choices and maintain a healthy weight before, during, and after treatment. A registered dietitian (RD) has at least a bachelor's degree and has passed a national competency exam.

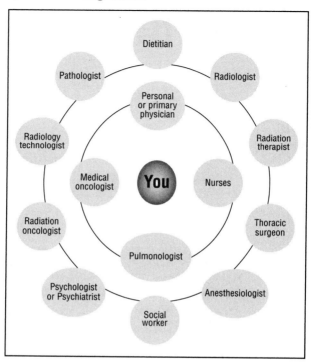

Medical Oncologist

A medical oncologist (also sometimes simply called an oncologist) is a medical doctor you may see after diagnosis. The oncologist is a cancer expert who understands specific types of cancer, their treatments, and their causes. He or she may help people with cancer make decisions about a course of treatment and then manage all phases of cancer care. Oncologists most often become involved when you need chemotherapy, but can also prescribe hormonal therapy and other anticancer drugs.

Nurses

During your treatment you will be in contact with different types of nurses.

Registered nurse

A registered nurse has an associate or bachelor's degree in nursing and has passed a state licensing exam. She or he can monitor your condition, provide treatment, educate you about side effects, and help you adjust to lung cancer physically and emotionally.

Nurse practitioner

A nurse practitioner is a registered nurse with a master's or doctoral degree who can manage lung cancer care and has additional training in primary care. He or she shares many tasks with your doctors, such as recording your medical history, conducting physical exams, and doing follow-up care. In most states, a nurse practitioner can prescribe medicines with a doctor's supervision.

Clinical nurse specialist

A clinical nurse specialist (CNS) is a nurse who has a master's degree in a specific area, such as oncology, psychiatry, or critical care nursing. The CNS often provides expertise to staff and may provide special services to patients, such as leading support groups and coordinating cancer care.

Oncology-certified nurse

An oncology-certified nurse is a clinical nurse who has demonstrated an in-depth knowledge of oncology care. He or she has passed a certification exam. Oncology-certified nurses are found in all areas of cancer practice.

Pathologist

A pathologist is a medical doctor specially trained in diagnosing disease based on the examination of microscopic tissue and fluid samples. He or she will determine the classification (cell type) of your cancer, help determine the stage (extent) and grade (estimate of aggressiveness) of your cancer, and issue a pathology report so that you and your doctor can decide on treatment options.

Personal or Primary Care Physician

A personal physician may be a general doctor, internist, or family practice doctor. He or she is often the medical doctor you first saw when you noticed symptoms of illness. This general or family practice doctor may be a member of your medical team, but a specialist is most often a patient's cancer care team leader.

Psychologist or Psychiatrist

A psychologist is a licensed mental health professional who is often part of the medical team. He or she provides counseling on emotional and psychological issues. A psychologist may have specialized training and experience treating people with cancer.

A psychiatrist is a medical doctor specializing in mental health and behavioral disorders. Psychiatrists provide counseling and can also prescribe medications.

Pulmonologist

A pulmonologist is a doctor who specializes in the diagnosis and treatment of lung diseases. A pulmonologist may have first diagnosed your lung cancer, and you may continue to see this doctor if you have breathing trouble related to the cancer or other lung problems.

Radiation Oncologist

A radiation oncologist is a medical doctor who specializes in treating cancer by using therapeutic radiation (high-energy x-rays or seeds). If you choose radiation, this member of your medical team evaluates you frequently during the course of treatment and at intervals afterward. The radiation oncologist will usually work closely with your oncologist. He or she helps you make decisions about radiation therapy options. A radiation oncologist is assisted by a radiation therapist during treatment and works with a radiation physicist, an expert who is trained in ensuring that the right dose of radiation treatment is delivered to you. The physicist is also assisted by a dosimetrist, a technician who helps plan and calculate the dosage, number, and length of your radiation treatments.

Radiation Therapist

A radiation therapist is a specially trained technician who works with the equipment that delivers radiation therapy. He or she positions your body during the treatment and administers the radiation therapy.

Radiologist

A radiologist is a medical doctor specializing in the use of imaging procedures (for example, diagnostic x-rays, ultrasound, magnetic resonance images, bone scans, and others) that produce pictures of internal body structures. He or she has special training in diagnosing cancer and other diseases and interpreting the results of imaging procedures. Your radiologist issues a radiology report describing the findings to your pulmonologist, medical oncologist, or radiation oncologist. The radiology images and report may be used to aid in diagnosis, to help classify and determine the extent of your lung cancer, to help locate tumors during procedures and radiation treatment, or to look for the possible spread or recurrence of the cancer after treatment.

Radiology Technologist

A radiology technologist is a trained health care professional who assists the radiologist by positioning your body for x-rays and other procedures and developing and checking the images for quality. The radiologist then reads these images.

Social Worker

A social worker is a health specialist, usually with a master's degree, who is licensed or certified by the state in which he or she works. A social worker is an expert in coordinating and providing social services. He or she is trained to help you and your family deal with a range of emotional and practical challenges, such as finances, child care, emotional issues, family concerns and relationships, transportation, and problems with the health care system. If your social worker is trained in cancer-related problems, he or she can counsel you about your fears or concerns, help answer questions about diagnosis and treatment, and lead cancer support groups. You may communicate with your social worker during a hospital stay or on an outpatient basis.

Thoracic Surgeon

A thoracic surgeon is a doctor who specializes in performing chest surgery. This doctor will most likely do any tumor biopsies that are part of the lung cancer diagnosis.

How Is Small Cell Lung Cancer Treated?

This information represents the views of the doctors and nurses serving on the American Cancer Society's Cancer Information Database Editorial Board. These views are based on their interpretation of studies published in medical journals, as well as their own professional experience.

The treatment information in this document is not official policy of the Society and is not intended as medical advice to replace the expertise and judgment of your cancer care team. It is intended to help you and your family make informed decisions, together with your doctor.

Your doctor may have reasons for suggesting a treatment plan different from these general treatment options. Don't hesitate to ask him or her questions about your treatment options.

If you have small cell lung cancer, your main treatment will be chemotherapy, either alone or in combination with radiation, and—very rarely—surgery, depending on the stage of your cancer.

After the cancer is found and staged, your cancer care team will discuss your treatment options with you. It is important to take time and think about all of your possible choices. In choosing a treatment plan, the most significant factors to consider are the type of cancer (small cell or non–small cell) and the stage of the cancer. For this reason, it is very important that your doctor order all the tests needed to determine the cancer's stage.

Other factors to consider include your overall physical health, **performance status**, likely **side effects** of the treatment, and the probability of curing the disease, extending life, or relieving symptoms. One thing to remember is that age alone should not be a barrier to treatment. Older people can benefit from treatment as much as younger people as long as their general health is good.

In considering your treatment options it is often a good idea to seek a second opinion. A second opinion may provide more information and help you feel more confident about the treatment plan you have chosen. Your doctor should not mind your doing this. In fact, some insurance companies require you to get a second opinion. If your first doctor has done tests, the results can be sent to the second doctor so that you will not have to have them done again. If you are in an HMO (health maintenance organization), find out about its policy concerning second opinions.

Surgery

Surgery is rarely used in small cell lung cancer. Occasionally (in about 1 out of 20 cases), the small cell lung cancer forms only one localized tumor nodule, with no spread to lymph nodes or other organs. Removal of the cancer is justified in these cases, and is usually followed by additional treatment (chemotherapy and radiation therapy).

If a section (lobe) of the lung is removed, the operation is called a **lobectomy**. If the entire lung is removed, the surgery is called a **pneumonectomy**. Removing part of a lobe is known as a **segmentectomy** or wedge **resection.**

These operations require general anesthesia (you are "asleep") and a surgical incision is made in the chest (called thoracotomy). You will generally spend 1 to 2 weeks in the hospital. Possible complications include excessive bleeding, wound infections, and pneumonia. Because the surgeon must spread ribs to get to the lung, the incision will hurt for some time after surgery. Your activity will be limited for at least a month or 2.

If your lungs are in good condition (other than the presence of the cancer) you can usually return to normal activities after a lobe or even an entire lung has been removed. However, if your lungs have been damaged and you have noncancerous diseases such as emphysema or chronic bronchitis (which are common among heavy smokers), you may become short of breath after surgery. Pulmonary function tests are done before surgery to determine whether you will have enough healthy lung tissue remaining after surgery.

If you can't undergo a thoracotomy because of lung disease or other serious medical problems, or if the cancer is widespread, other types of surgery can be used to relieve some symptoms. For example, laser surgery can be used to relieve blockage of airways that may be causing pneumonia or shortness of breath.

Recently, a less invasive procedure for treating early stage lung cancer has been developed. This is called video-assisted thoracic surgery. A small hollow tube with a video camera attached to the end can be placed through a small hole in the chest to help the surgeon see the tumor. Only small incisions are needed, so there is a little less pain after the surgery. Most experts recommend that only tumors smaller than 3 to 4 cm (about 1½ inches) be treated this way. The cure rate after this surgery seems to be the same as with older techniques. It is important, though, that the surgeon performing this procedure be experienced since it requires more technical skill than the standard surgery. An advantage of this surgery is a shorter hospital stay, usually around 5 days.

Sometimes fluid accumulates in the chest cavity and interferes with breathing. In order to remove the fluid and keep it from coming back, doctors will perform a procedure called **pleurodesis**. A small tube is placed in the chest, all the fluid removed, and either talc or a drug such as tetracycline or a chemotherapy drug is instilled into the chest cavity. These cause irritation and scarring that will seal the space and prevent fluid buildup. The tube is generally left in a day or two to drain any new fluid that might accumulate.

Radiation Therapy

Radiation therapy uses high-energy rays (such as x-rays) to kill cancer cells.

External beam radiation therapy uses radiation delivered from outside the body that is focused on the cancer. In limited stage small cell lung cancer it is most frequently used in addition to chemotherapy to treat the tumor and lymph nodes in the chest.

After chemotherapy, radiation therapy can be used to kill very small deposits of cancer that have not been eliminated. Radiation therapy can also be used to relieve symptoms of lung cancer such as pain, bleeding, difficulty swallowing, cough, and problems caused by brain metastases. It is usually given in small daily doses over several weeks.

Side effects of radiation therapy might include mild skin problems, nausea, vomiting, and **fatigue**. Often these go away after a short while. Radiation might also make the side effects of chemotherapy worse. Chest radiation therapy may damage your lungs and cause difficulty breathing and shortness of breath. Your esophagus, which is located in the middle of your chest, will be exposed to radiation. For this reason, you might have difficulty swallowing during the treatment. This will improve after treatment is over.

Radiation therapy is often given prophylactically to the brain in limited SCLC since the brain is a common site of metastasis. Radiation therapy to large areas of the brain can sometimes change your brain function. You may notice memory loss, headache, difficulty thinking, or diminished sexual desire. Usually these symptoms are minor compared to those caused by a brain tumor; nevertheless, they can reduce your quality of life. Side effects of radiation therapy to the brain usually become most serious 1 or 2 years after treatment.

Chemotherapy

Chemotherapy is treatment with anticancer drugs given into a vein or by mouth. These drugs enter the bloodstream and reach throughout the body, making this treatment useful for cancer that has spread or metastasized to organs beyond the lung. Chemotherapy is usually the main treatment for SCLC.

Chemotherapy for SCLC generally uses a combination of anticancer drugs. Doctors who prescribe these drugs (medical oncologists) generally use a combination of medicines that have proven to be more effective than a single drug. Doctors give chemotherapy in cycles, with each period of treatment followed by a recovery period. Chemotherapy cycles generally last about 21 to 28 days, and initial treatment typically involves 4 to 6 cycles. Chemotherapy is not recommended for patients in poor health (performance status 3–4). Advanced age is not a barrier, as long as the patient is not in poor health.

The drug combinations most frequently used for initial chemotherapy for SCLC are these:

- Limited Stage
  - Cisplatin and etoposide
  - Carboplatin and etoposide
- Extensive Stage
  - Cisplatin and etoposide
  - Carboplatin and etoposide
  - Cisplatin and irinotecan

These chemotherapy drugs are used if there has been a **relapse** of the SCLC:

- Ifosfamide, paclitaxel, docetaxel, or gemcitabine, if the relapse occurred within 2 to 3 months.
- Topotecan, irinotecan, cyclophosphamide/doxorubicin/vincristine (CAV), gemcitabine, paclitaxel, docetaxel, oral etoposide, methotrexate, or vinorelbine, if the relapse occurred from 2 to 3 months to 6 months.
- For relapses after 6 months, the original chemotherapy can be repeated.

Chemotherapy drugs kill cancer cells but also damage some normal cells. Therefore, your doctors will pay careful attention to avoiding or minimizing side effects. These depend on the type of drugs, the amount taken, and the length of treatment. Temporary side effects might include nausea and vomiting, loss of appetite, loss of hair, and mouth sores. Some drugs cause severe diarrhea.

Because chemotherapy can damage the blood-producing cells of the bone marrow, you may have low blood cell counts. Low blood cell counts can increase your risk for the following:

- infection (due to a shortage of white blood cells)
- bleeding or bruising after minor cuts or injuries (due to a shortage of blood platelets)
- fatigue or shortness of breath (due to low red blood cell counts)

Since cisplatin, vinorelbine, docetaxel, or paclitaxel can damage nerves, you might feel numbness and tingling, particularly in your fingers and toes, and sometimes your arms and legs might feel weak (this is called peripheral neuropathy). You should report this, as well as any other side effects or changes you experience while getting chemotherapy, to your medical team.

Some side effects disappear within a few days after treatment. There are remedies for many of these temporary side effects of chemotherapy. For example, your doctor can prescribe drugs for you to prevent or lessen nausea and vomiting.

Clinical Trials

The purpose of clinical trials

Studies of promising new or experimental treatments in patients are known as clinical trials. A clinical trial is only done when there is some reason to believe that the treatment being studied may be valuable to the patient. Treatments used in clinical trials are often found to have real benefits. Researchers conduct studies of new treatments to answer the following questions:

- Is the treatment helpful?
- How does this new type of treatment work?

- Does it work better than other treatments already available?
- What side effects does the treatment cause?
- Are the side effects greater or less than the **standard therapy**?
- Do the benefits outweigh the side effects?
- In which patients is the treatment most likely to be helpful?

Types of clinical trials

There are 3 phases of clinical trials in which a treatment is studied before it is eligible for approval by the Food and Drug Administration (FDA).

Phase I clinical trials

The purpose of a phase I study is to find the best way to give a new treatment and how much of it can be given safely. The cancer care team watches patients carefully for any harmful side effects. The treatment has been well tested in lab and animal studies, but the side effects in patients are not completely known. Doctors conducting the clinical trial start by giving very low doses of the drug to the first patients and increasing the dose for later groups of patients until side effects appear. Although doctors are hoping to help patients, the main purpose of a phase I study is to test the safety of the drug.

Phase II clinical trials

These studies are designed to see if the drug works. Patients are given the highest dose that doesn't cause severe side effects (determined from the phase I study) and closely observed for an effect on the cancer. The cancer care team also looks for side effects.

Phase III clinical trials

Phase III studies involve large numbers of patients—often several hundred. One group (the **control group**) receives the standard (most accepted) treatment. The other group receives the new treatment. All patients in phase III studies are closely watched. The study will be stopped if the side effects of the new treatment are too severe or if one group has had much better results than the others.

If you are in a clinical trial, you will have a team of experts taking care of you and monitoring your progress very carefully. The study is especially designed to pay close attention to you.

However, there are some risks. No one involved in the study knows in advance whether the treatment will work or exactly what side effects will occur. That is what the study is designed to find out. While most side effects disappear in time, some can be permanent or even life threatening. Keep in mind, though, that even standard treatments have side effects. Depending on many factors, you may decide to enroll in a clinical trial.

Deciding to enter a clinical trial

Enrollment in any clinical trial is completely up to you. Your doctors and nurses will explain the study to you in detail and will give you a form to read and sign indicating your desire to take part. This process is known as giving your **informed**

consent. Even after signing the form and after the clinical trial begins, you are free to leave the study at any time, for any reason. Taking part in the study does not prevent you from getting other medical care you may need.

To find out more about clinical trials, ask your cancer care team. The following are among the questions you should ask:

- Is there a clinical trial for which I would be eligible?
- What is the purpose of the study?
- What kinds of tests and treatments does the study involve?
- What does this treatment do? Has it been used before?
- Will I know which treatment I receive?
- What is likely to happen in my case with, or without, this new treatment?
- What are my other choices and their advantages and disadvantages?
- How could the study affect my daily life?
- What side effects can I expect from the study? Can the side effects be controlled?
- Will I have to be hospitalized? If so, how often and for how long?
- Will the study cost me anything? Will any of the treatment be free?
- If I am harmed as a result of the research, what treatment would I be entitled to?
- What type of long-term follow-up care is part of the study?
- Has the treatment been used to treat other types of cancers?

The American Cancer Society offers a clinical trials matching service for patients, their family, and friends. You can access this service on our Web site at http://clinicaltrials.cancer.org or by calling 1-800-303-5691. Based on the information you provide about your cancer type, stage, and previous treatments, this service can compile a list of clinical trials that match your medical needs. In finding a center most convenient for you, the service can also take into account where you live and whether you are willing to travel.

You can also get a list of current clinical trials by calling the National Cancer Institute's Cancer Information Service toll free at 1-800-4-CANCER or by visiting the NCI clinical trials Web site at www.cancer.gov/clinical_trials/.

Complementary and Alternative Therapies

Complementary and alternative therapies are a diverse group of health care practices, systems, and products that are not part of usual medical treatment. They may include products such as vitamins, herbs, or **dietary supplements**, or procedures such as acupuncture, massage, and a host of other types of treatment. There is a great deal of interest today in complementary and alternative treatments for cancer. Many are now being studied to find out if they are truly helpful to people with cancer.

You may hear about different treatments from family, friends, and others, which may be offered as a way to treat your cancer or to help you feel better. Some of these treatments are harmless in certain situations, while others have been shown to cause harm. Most of them are of unproven benefit.

The American Cancer Society defines **complementary therapy** or methods as those that are used along with your regular medical care. If these treatments are carefully managed, they may add to your comfort and well-being. **Alternative therapy** or methods are defined as those that are used instead of your regular medical care. Some of them have been proven not to be useful or even to be harmful, but are still promoted as "cures." If you choose to use these alternatives, they may reduce your chance of fighting your cancer by delaying, replacing, or interfering with regular cancer treatment.

Treatment Choices for Small Cell Lung Cancer

If you smoke, it is important that you try to quit. Studies have shown that patients who continue to smoke after the diagnosis of lung cancer have worse outcomes than those who stop.

This type of cancer is usually staged as either limited or extensive. Studies show that this type of lung cancer has usually spread by the time it is found (even if that spread is not shown by x-rays and other imaging tests), so SCLC usually cannot be treated by surgery alone.

Limited stage

If you have limited stage SCLC you will receive chemotherapy. If you only have a single nodule in your lung and no evidence of cancer elsewhere, your doctors may recommend that the tumor and mediastinal lymph nodes first be surgically removed. After that, you will receive chemotherapy, with or without radiation. The most commonly used treatment is a combination of 2 or more chemotherapy drugs. These will be either cisplatin or carboplatin combined with etoposide, usually given for around 6 months. Clinical trials are being done to see whether adding topotecan or paclitaxel will improve survival.

Many studies have been done to find out whether radiation treatment to the chest (usually the middle where the cancer spreads to lymph nodes) will improve your survival chances better than chemotherapy alone. These studies have shown that radiation does provide benefit, particularly when done early. Radiation is recommended if cancer is found in the lymph nodes that were removed. The radiation is often given along with the chemotherapy. Although this increases the side effects of treatment, it appears to be more effective than delaying either the radiation or chemotherapy. You may have more trouble breathing because of lung damage and also may have trouble swallowing because your esophagus can be affected by the radiation.

You will not be given chest radiation therapy if you have another severe lung disease (in addition to your cancer) or other types of serious health problems.

If you are treated with chemotherapy, with or without radiation therapy, it is likely that your tumor will shrink and you will go into **remission**. Sooner or later, though, your cancer may begin to grow again.

Extensive stage

If you have extensive SCLC, chemotherapy can treat your symptoms and also allow you to live longer. Your treatment will depend on exactly where your cancer has spread and will also be influenced by your general state of health. The chance of your cancer shrinking with chemotherapy is about 70% to 80%. Once again, carboplatin or cisplatin along with etoposide are the usual drugs given. Some doctors favor giving large doses of chemotherapy along with drugs that build up the blood cell count (colony-stimulating factors). It still isn't clear whether this approach improves the results of chemotherapy.

However, the cancer eventually becomes resistant to the chemotherapy. A second type of chemotherapy can be given and some people will respond to this, although usually for only a short time. These drugs can include cyclophosphamide, doxorubicin, vincristine, ifosfamide, topotecan, paclitaxel, methotrexate, vinorelbine, gemcitabine, irinotecan and docetaxel in various combinations. Radiation therapy is sometimes used to control symptoms of cancer growth within the lung or spread to the bones or brain.

If your general health is very poor, you may not be able to withstand the side effects of chemotherapy or benefit from it. In this case, your doctor may select a treatment plan based on your individual medical situation. If you are too ill to have chemotherapy, the best plan may be to have supportive or **palliative treatment**, perhaps through a **hospice** program. This would include treatment of any pain, breathing problems, or other symptoms you might have. Pain can be a major problem if you have extensive lung cancer. Growth of the cancer around certain nerves may cause severe pain. However, medicine can effectively relieve this pain. Radiation therapy may also be helpful. It is important that you take advantage of these treatments.

Even if you have incurable lung cancer, you should try to get the most out of your life by making every day count. That means that you should be as free of symptoms as possible. You might consider a clinical trial of new chemotherapy drugs or other new treatments such as one that stops the formation of new blood vessels (**angiogenesis**); substances that interfere with growth factor action, or other related drugs; **immunotherapy**; or **gene therapy**. These are worthwhile options that may benefit you as well as future patients. Deciding on the right time to discontinue chemotherapy and focus on palliative care is never easy. Good communication with doctors, nurses, family, and clergy, as well as discussions with hospice staff, can help people facing this situation.

Adjuvant Treatment

SCLC commonly spreads to the brain. If no preventive measures are taken, about 50% of people with SCLC will have metastasis to their brain. For this reason, if you have responded well to initial treatment, you may be given brain radiation therapy to prevent brain metastasis. This is usually given in lower doses than that for treatment of known metastases.

One problem that doctors have reported is that some patients given preventive brain radiation may suffer side effects, such as trouble with memory and clumsiness. It is not totally clear that these symptoms are a direct result of the radiation. Most doctors will recommend brain radiation therapy if you have had a complete response (all the apparent cancer is gone) or the tumor has shrunk to less than 10% of its original size after chemotherapy. Studies have shown that preventive brain radiation has an overall survival advantage.

Recurrence of Limited Stage Disease

If your cancer has come back after chemotherapy, new chemotherapy can still help. You will be given drugs like those suggested for people with extensive disease. You may also consider a clinical trial or supportive care for symptom management.

More Treatment Information

For more details on treatment options—including some that may not be addressed in this book—the National Comprehensive Cancer Network (NCCN) and the National Cancer Institute (NCI) are good sources of information.

The NCCN, made up of experts from 20 of the nation's leading cancer centers, develops cancer treatment guidelines for doctors to use when treating patients. These are available on the NCCN Web site (www.nccn.org).

The American Cancer Society collaborates with the NCCN to produce a version of some of these treatment guidelines, written specifically for patients and their families. These less-technical versions are available on both the NCCN Web site (www.nccn.org) and the ACS Web site (www.cancer.org). A print version can also be requested from the ACS at 1-800-ACS-2345.

The NCI provides treatment guidelines via its telephone information center (1-800-4-CANCER) and its Web site (www.cancer.gov). Detailed guidelines intended for use by cancer care professionals are also available on www.cancer.gov.

Questions To Ask

What Should You Ask Your Doctor About Small Cell Lung Cancer?

It is important for you to have honest, open discussions with your cancer care team. They want to answer all of your questions, no matter how trivial you might think they are.

- ❑ What kind of lung cancer do I have?
- ❑ Has my cancer spread beyond the primary site?
- ❑ What is the stage of my cancer and what does that mean in my case?
- ❑ What treatment choices do I have?
- ❑ What do you recommend and why?
- ❑ What is my expected survival rate, based on my cancer as you see it?
- ❑ What risks or side effects are there to the treatments you suggest?
- ❑ What are the chances of recurrence of my cancer with these treatment plans?
- ❑ What should I do to be ready for treatment?

In addition to these sample questions, be sure to write down some of your own. For instance, you might want more information about recovery times so you can plan your work schedule. Or, you may want to ask about second opinions or about clinical trials for which you may qualify.

After Treatment

What Happens After Treatment for Small Cell Lung Cancer?

Completing treatment can be both stressful and exciting. You will be relieved to finish treatment, yet it is hard not to worry about cancer coming back. This is a very common concern among those who have had cancer.

It may take a while before your confidence in your own recovery begins to feel real and your fears are somewhat relieved. You can learn more about what to look for and how to learn to live with the possibility of cancer coming back in the American Cancer Society document *Living with Uncertainty: The Fear of Cancer Recurrence*, available at 1-800-ACS-2345.

Follow-up Care

After your treatment is over, it is very important to keep all follow-up appointments. During these visits, your doctors will ask about symptoms, do physical exams, and order blood tests or imaging tests such as CT scans or x-rays. Follow-up is needed to check for cancer **recurrence** or spread, as well as possible side effects of certain treatments. This is the time for you to ask your health care team any questions you need answered and to discuss any concerns you might have.

Almost any cancer treatment can have side effects. Some may last for a few weeks to several months, but others can be permanent. It is important for you to report any new or recurring symptoms to your doctor right away so that any problems related to a recurrent cancer or side effects of treatment can be dealt with promptly.

It is also important to keep medical insurance. Even though no one wants to think of their cancer coming back, it is always a possibility. If it happens, the last thing you want is to have to worry about paying for treatment. Many people have been bankrupted by cancer recurrence. Should your cancer come back, the American Cancer Society document *When Your Cancer Comes Back: Cancer Recurrence* gives you information on how to manage and cope with this phase of your treatment. You can get this document by calling 1-800-ACS-2345.

Seeing a New Doctor

At some point after your cancer diagnosis and treatment, you may find yourself in the office of a new doctor. Your original doctor may have moved or retired, or you may have moved or changed doctors for some reason. It is important that you be able to give your new doctor the exact details of your diagnosis and treatment. Make sure you have the following information handy:

- a copy of your pathology report from any biopsy or surgery
- if you had surgery, a copy of your operative report
- if you were hospitalized, a copy of the discharge summary that every doctor must prepare when patients are sent home from the hospital
- finally, since some drugs can have long-term side effects, a list of your drugs, drug doses, and when you took them

After you show this to your new doctor, get your copies back and keep them in a safe place. You will likely need them again and again.

Lifestyle Changes to Consider During and After Treatment

Having cancer and dealing with treatment can be time-consuming and emotionally draining, but it can also be a time to look at your life in new ways. Maybe you are thinking about how to improve your health over the long term. Some people even begin this process during cancer treatment.

Make Healthier Choices

Think about your life before you learned you had cancer. Were there things you did that might have made you less healthy? Maybe you drank too much alcohol, or ate more than you needed, or smoked, or didn't exercise very often. Emotionally, maybe you kept your feelings bottled up, or maybe you let stressful situations go on too long.

Now is not the time to feel guilty or to blame yourself. However, you can start making changes *today* that can have positive effects for the rest of your life. Not only will you feel better but you will also be healthier. What better time than *now* to take advantage of the motivation you have as a result of going through a life-changing experience like having cancer?

You can start by working on those things that you feel most concerned about. Get help with those that are harder for you. For instance, if you are thinking about quitting smoking and need help, call the American Cancer Society's Quitline® tobacco cessation program at 1-800-ACS-2345.

Diet and Nutrition

Eating right can be a challenge for anyone, but it can get even tougher during and after cancer treatment. For instance, treatment often may change your sense of taste. Nausea can be a problem. You may lose your appetite for a while and lose weight when you don't want to. On the other hand, some people gain weight even without eating more. This can be frustrating too.

If you are losing weight or have taste problems during treatment, do the best you can with eating and remember that these problems usually improve over time. You may want to ask your cancer team for a referral to a dietitian, an expert in nutrition who can give you ideas on how to manage some of the side effects of your treatment. You may also find it helps to eat small portions every 2 to 3 hours until you feel better and can go back to a more normal schedule.

One of the best things you can do after treatment is to put healthy eating habits into place. You will be surprised at the long-term benefits of some simple changes, like increasing the variety of healthy foods you eat. Try to eat 5 or more servings of vegetables and fruits each day. Choose whole grain foods instead of white flour and sugars. Try to limit meats that are high in fat. Cut back on processed meats like hot dogs, bologna, and bacon. Get rid of them altogether if you can. If you drink alcohol, limit yourself to 1 or 2 drinks a day at the most. And don't forget to get some type of regular exercise. The combination of a good diet and regular exercise will help you maintain a healthy weight and keep you feeling more energetic.

Rest, Fatigue, Work, and Exercise

Fatigue is a very common symptom in people being treated for cancer. This is often not an ordinary type of tiredness but a "bone-weary" exhaustion that doesn't get better with rest. For some, this fatigue lasts a long time after treatment, and can discourage them from physical activity.

However, exercise can actually help you reduce fatigue. Studies have shown that patients who follow an exercise program tailored to their personal needs feel physically and emotionally improved and can cope better.

If you are ill and need to be on bed rest during treatment, it is normal to expect your fitness, endurance, and muscle strength to decline some.

Physical therapy can help you maintain strength and range of motion in your muscles, which can help fight fatigue and the sense of depression that sometimes comes with feeling so tired.

Any program of physical activity should fit your own situation. An older person who has never exercised will not be able to take on the same amount of exercise as a 20-year-old who plays tennis 3 times a week. If you haven't exercised in a few years but can still get around, you may want to think about taking short walks.

Talk with your health care team before starting, and get their opinion about your exercise plans. Then, try to get an exercise buddy so that you're not doing it alone. Having family or friends involved when starting a new exercise program can give you that extra boost of support to keep you going when the push just isn't there.

If you are very tired, though, you will need to balance activity with rest. It is okay to rest when you need to. It is really hard for some people to allow themselves to do that when they are used to working all day or taking care of a household. (For more information about fatigue, please see the publication *Cancer-Related Fatigue and Anemia Treatment Guidelines for Patients*.

Exercise can improve both your physical and emotional health:

- It improves your cardiovascular (heart and circulation) fitness.
- It strengthens your muscles.
- It reduces fatigue.

- It lowers anxiety and depression.
- It makes you feel generally happier.
- It helps you feel better about yourself.

And long term, we know that exercise plays a role in preventing some cancers. The American Cancer Society, in its guidelines on physical activity for cancer **prevention**, recommends that adults take part in at least 1 physical activity for 30 minutes or more on 5 days or more of the week. Children and teens are encouraged to try for at least 60 minutes a day of energetic physical activity on at least 5 days a week.

How About Your Emotional Health?

Once your treatment ends, you may find yourself overwhelmed by emotions. This happens to a lot of people. You may have been going through so much during treatment that you could only focus on getting through your treatment.

Now you may find that you think about the potential of your own death, or the effect of your cancer on your family, friends, and career. You may also begin to re-evaluate your relationship with your spouse or partner. Unexpected issues may also cause concern—for instance, as you become healthier and have fewer doctor visits, you will see your health care team less often. That can be a source of anxiety for some.

This is an ideal time to seek out emotional and social support. You need people you can turn to for strength and comfort. Support can come in many forms: family, friends, cancer support groups, church or spiritual groups, online support communities, or individual counselors.

Almost everyone who has been through cancer can benefit from getting some type of support. What's best for you depends on your situation and personality. Some people feel safe in peer-support groups or education groups. Others would rather talk in an informal setting, such as church. Others may feel more at ease talking one-on-one with a trusted friend or counselor. Whatever your source of strength or comfort, make sure you have a place to go with your concerns.

The cancer journey can feel very lonely. It is not necessary or realistic to go it all by yourself. And your friends and family may feel shut out if you decide not to include them. Let them in—and let in anyone else who you feel may help. If you aren't sure who can help, call your American Cancer Society at 1-800-ACS-2345 and we can put you in touch with an appropriate group or resource.

You can't change the fact that you have had cancer. What you can change is how you live the rest of your life—making healthy choices and feeling as well as possible, physically and emotionally.

What Happens if Treatment Is No Longer Working?

If cancer continues to grow after one kind of treatment, or if it returns, it is often possible to try another treatment plan that might still cure the cancer, or at least shrink the tumors enough to help you live longer and feel better. On the other hand, when a person has received several different medical treatments and the cancer has not fully responded, over time the cancer tends to become resistant to all treatment. At this time, it's important to weigh the possible limited benefit of a new treatment against the possible downsides, including continued doctor visits and treatment side effects.

Everyone has his or her own way of looking at this. Some people may want to focus on remaining comfortable during their limited time left.

This is likely to be the most difficult time in your battle with cancer—when you have tried everything medically within reason and it's just not working anymore. Although your doctor may offer you new treatment, you need to consider that at some point, continuing treatment is not likely to improve your health or change your prognosis.

If you want to continue treatment to fight your cancer as long as you can, you still need to consider the odds of more treatment having any benefit. In many cases, your doctor can estimate the response rate for the treatment you are considering. Some people are tempted to try more chemotherapy or radiation, for example, even when their doctors say that the odds of benefit are less than 1%. In this situation, you need to think about and understand your reasons for choosing this plan.

No matter what you decide to do, it is important that you be as comfortable as possible. Make sure you are asking for and getting treatment for any symptoms you might have, such as pain. This type of treatment is called palliative treatment.

Palliative treatment helps relieve these symptoms, but is not expected to cure the disease; its main purpose is to improve your quality of life. Sometimes, the treatments you get to control your symptoms are similar to the treatments used to treat cancer. For example, radiation therapy might be given to help relieve bone pain from bone metastasis. Or chemotherapy might be given to help shrink a tumor and keep it from causing a bowel obstruction. But this is not the same as receiving treatment to try to cure the cancer.

At some point, you may benefit from hospice care. Most of the time, this can be given at home. Your cancer may be causing symptoms or problems that need attention, and hospice focuses on your comfort. You should know that receiving hospice care doesn't mean you can't have treatment for the problems caused by your cancer or other health conditions. It just means that the focus of your care is on living life as fully as possible and feeling as well as you can at this difficult stage of your cancer.

Remember that maintaining hope is also important. Your hope for a cure may not be as bright, but there is still hope for good times with family and friends—times that are filled with happiness and meaning. In a way, pausing at this time in your cancer treatment is an opportunity to refocus on the most important things in your life. This is the time to do some things you've always wanted to do and to stop doing the things you no longer want to do.

Latest Research

What's New in Small Cell Lung Cancer Research and Treatment?

Progress in prevention, early detection, and treatment based on current research is expected to save many thousands of lives each year. Lung cancer research is currently being done in medical centers throughout the world.

Prevention

At this time, many researchers believe that prevention offers the greatest opportunity to fight lung cancer. Although decades have passed since the link between smoking and lung cancers was clearly identified, scientists estimate that smoking is still responsible for about 85%–90% of lung cancers. Research is continuing in these areas:

- ways to help people quit smoking through counseling, nicotine replacement, and other medications
- ways to convince young people to never start smoking

- identifying inherited differences in genes that may make some people exceptionally likely to get lung cancer if they smoke or are exposed to someone else's smoke

Although researchers are looking for ways to use vitamins or medicine to prevent lung cancer in people at high risk, these have so far not proved successful. For now most researchers think that simply following the American Cancer Society dietary recommendations (such as choosing most foods from plant sources and eating at least 5 servings of fruits and vegetables each day) may be the best strategy.

Earlier Diagnosis

Nearly 20 years ago, large studies were done to determine whether routine chest x-rays and sputum cytology testing could save lives. Most researchers concluded that these tests did not find lung cancers early enough to significantly lower the risk of death from lung cancer. However, some researchers disagree about the best way to interpret the studies' data and the debate continues.

A large clinical trial called the National Lung Screening Trial (NLST) is underway to test whether spiral CT scanning of people at high risk of lung cancer will save lives. Information from this study will be coming out in the next few years. (For more information about the NLST, ask the American Cancer Society or the National Cancer Institute.) Another approach uses new ways to more sensitively detect cancer cells in sputum samples.

Researchers have recently found several changes that often affect the DNA of lung cancer cells. Current studies are evaluating new diagnostic tests that specifically recognize these DNA changes to see if this approach is useful in finding lung cancers at an earlier stage.

Treatment

Chemotherapy

Doctors are using newer chemotherapy drugs more often in place of the older ones with more serious side effects. Studies are also testing the best ways to combine chemotherapy with radiation therapy and to decrease the side effects of certain chemotherapy drugs.

Gene therapy

Great advances have been made over the past 20 years in understanding how DNA changes cause cells to become cancerous and how DNA regulates the immune system's response to cancer cells. Many researchers believe this progress can be applied to develop more effective ways of treating lung cancer through gene therapy.

Researchers are developing ways to alter lung cancers by adding extra DNA so that cancer cells are better recognized and more effectively attacked by the patient's immune system. They are using DNA to repair the gene mutations thought to be responsible for the lung cell's original transformation into a cancer cell.

Antiangiogenesis drugs

In order for cancers to grow, blood vessels must develop to nourish the cancer cells. This process is called angiogenesis. New drugs that inhibit angiogenesis are under investigation as lung cancer treatments. Some have already been successfully used for other cancer types. A new drug called bevacizumab has shown some benefit in clinical trials of patients with NSCLC, and is currently being tested in small cell lung cancer. Other new drugs are being developed that may also be useful in stopping lung cancer growth by preventing new blood vessels from forming. Several of these drugs are being tested in clinical trials and trials of new, more potent, antiangiogenesis drugs are expected to begin soon.

Vaccines

Many studies that try to get the body's immune system to fight the cancer are in progress. In general these will be most effective in patients with early stage cancer, perhaps after surgery.

Resources

Additional Resources

More Information from Your American Cancer Society

The following related information may also be helpful to you. These materials may be ordered from our toll-free number, 1-800-ACS-2345.

After Diagnosis: A Guide for Patients and Families (also available in Spanish)

Caring for the Person with Cancer at Home: A Guide for Patients and Families (also available in Spanish)

Pain Control: A Guide for People With Cancer and Their Families (also available in Spanish)

Questions About Smoking, Tobacco, and Health (also available in Spanish)

Understanding Chemotherapy (also available in Spanish)

Understanding Radiation Therapy (also available in Spanish)

The following books are available from the American Cancer Society. Call us at 1-800-ACS-2345 to ask about costs or to place your order.

American Cancer Society Consumer Guide to Cancer Drugs, Second Edition

American Cancer Society's Complementary and Alternative Cancer Methods Handbook

*American Cancer Society's Guide to Pain Control:
Understanding and Managing Cancer Pain*,
Revised Edition

Because... Someone I Love Has Cancer: Kids' Activity Book

*Cancer in the Family: Helping Children Cope with a
Parent's Illness*

Cancer: What Causes It, What Doesn't

*Caregiving: A Step-By-Step Resource for Caring for the
Person with Cancer at Home*, Revised Edition

*Coming to Terms with Cancer: A Glossary of Cancer-
Related Terms*

*Couples Confronting Cancer: Keeping Your
Relationship Strong*

Eating Well, Staying Well: During and After Cancer

*Informed Decisions: The Complete Book of Cancer
Diagnosis, Treatment, and Recovery*, Second Edition

*Kicking Butts: Quit Smoking and Take Charge of
Your Health*

*Lymphedema: Understanding and Managing Lymphedema
After Cancer Treatment*

Our Mom Has Cancer

When the Focus Is on Care: Palliative Care and Cancer

National Organizations and Web Sites*

In addition to the American Cancer Society, other
sources of patient information and support
include:

American Lung Association
Telephone: 1-800-586-4872
Internet address: www.lungusa.org

It's Time To Focus On Lung Cancer
Telephone: 1-877-646-LUNG (1-877-646-5864)
Internet address: www.lungcancer.org

Lung Cancer Alliance
Telephone: 1-800-298-2436 (United States only)
or 1-202-463-2080
Internet address: www.lungcanceralliance.org

National Cancer Institute
Telephone: 1-800-4-CANCER (1-800-422-6237)
Internet address: www.cancer.gov

*Inclusion on this list does not imply endorsement by the American Cancer Society

The American Cancer Society is happy to address almost any cancer-related topic. If you have any more questions, please call us at 1-800-ACS-2345, any time, any day.

References

American Cancer Society. *Cancer Facts and Figures 2007*. Atlanta, Ga: American Cancer Society; 2007.

American Joint Committee on Cancer. Lung. *AJCC Cancer Staging Manual*. 6th ed. New York: Springer. 167-177.

Jackman DM, Johnson BE. Small-cell lung cancer. *Lancet* 2005;366:1385-1396.

Murren J, Turrisi AT, Pass HI. Small cell lung cancer. In: DeVita VT, Heilman S, Rosenberg SA, eds. *Cancer: Principles and Practice of Oncology*. 7th ed. Philadelphia, Pa: Lippincott Williams & Wilkins 2005: 810-844.

NCCN Clinical Practice Guidelines in Oncology. Small Cell Lung Cancer. Version 1, 2006. www.nccn.org. Accessed August 2006.

Ruckdeschel JC, Schwartz AG, Bepler G, et al. Cancer of the lung: NSCLC and SCLC. In: Abeloff MD, Armitage JO, Lichter AS, Niederhuber JE. Kastan MB, McKenna WG. *Clinical Oncology*. 3rd ed. Philadelphia, Pa. Elsevier: 2004:1649-1743.

U.S. Preventive Services Task Force. Lung cancer screening. *Ann Intern Med*. 2004;140:738-739.

Vaporciyan AA, Kiesw M,, Stevens CW, Komaki R, Roth JA. Cancer of the lung. In: Kufe DW, Pollock RE, Weichselbaum RR, Bast RC, Gansler TS, Holland JF, Frei E. *Cancer Medicine 6*. Hamilton, Ont: BC Decker; 2003. 1385-1446

Dictionary

adenocarcinoma (add-en-o-kahr-si-NO-muh): cancer that starts in the glandular tissue, such as in the ducts or lobules of the breast or the outer region of the lungs.

adjuvant therapy (ADD-joo-vunt therapy): treatment used in addition to the main treatment. It usually refers to hormonal therapy, chemotherapy, radiation therapy, or immunotherapy added after surgery to increase the chances of curing the disease or keeping it in check.

advanced stage: a general term describing cancer that has spread from the primary site to other parts of the body. When the cancer has spread only to the surrounding areas, it is called locally or regionally advanced. If it has spread to distant parts of the body, it is called metastatic. *See* primary site.

alternative therapy: an unproven therapy that is recommended instead of standard (proven) therapy. Some alternative therapies have dangerous or even life-threatening side effects. With others, the main danger is that the patient may lose the opportunity to benefit from standard therapy. The American Cancer Society recommends that patients considering the use of any alternative or complementary therapy discuss this with their health care team. *See also* complementary therapy, unproven therapy, and standard therapy.

alveoli (al-VEE-o-lie): air sacs of the lungs.

American Joint Committee on Cancer (AJCC) staging system: a system for describing the extent of a cancer's spread using Roman numerals from 0 through IV. Also called the TNM system. *See also* staging.

anemia (uh-NEEM-ee-uh): low red blood cell count.

anesthesia (an-es-THEE-zhuh): the loss of feeling or sensation as a result of drugs or gases. General anesthesia causes loss of consciousness ("puts you to sleep"). Local or regional anesthesia numbs only a certain area.

angiogenesis (an-jee-o-JEN-uh-sis): the formation of new blood vessels. Some cancer treatments work by blocking angiogenesis, thus preventing blood from reaching the tumor.

atypical (a-TIP-uh-kul): not usual; abnormal. Often refers to the appearance of cancerous or precancerous cells.

benign tumor: an abnormal growth that is not cancer and does not spread to other areas of the body.

biopsy: the removal of a sample of tissue to see whether cancer cells are present. There are several kinds of biopsies. In some, a very thin needle is used to draw fluid and cells from a lump. In a core biopsy, a larger needle is used to remove more tissue. *See also* CT–guided needle biopsy, needle biopsy, and needle aspiration.

blood count: a count of the number of red blood cells and white blood cells in a given sample of blood.

brachytherapy (brake-ee-THER-uh-pee): internal radiation treatment given by placing radioactive material directly into the tumor or close to it. Also called interstitial radiation therapy or seed implantation. *See* internal radiation. *Compare to* external beam radiation therapy.

bronchi (BRONG-ki): in the lungs, the 2 main air passages leading from the windpipe (trachea). The bronchi provide a passage for air to move in and out of the lungs.

bronchiole (BRONG-key-ol): one of the smaller sub-divisions of the bronchi.

bronchoscopy (brong-KOS-ko-pee): examination of the bronchi using a flexible, lighted tube called a bronchoscope.

cancer: cancer is not just one disease but a group of diseases. All forms of cancer cause cells in the body to change and grow out of control. Most types of cancer cells form a lump or mass called a tumor. The tumor can invade and destroy healthy tissue. Cells from the tumor can break away and travel to other parts of the body. There they can continue to grow. This spreading process is called metastasis. When cancer spreads, it is still named after the part of the body where it started. For example, if breast cancer spreads to the lungs, it is still breast cancer, not lung cancer.

Some cancers, such as blood cancers, do not form a tumor. Not all tumors are cancer. A tumor that is not cancer is called benign. Benign tumors do not grow and spread the way cancer does. They are usually not a threat to life. Another word for cancerous is malignant.

cancer care team: the group of health care professionals who work together to find, treat, and care for people with cancer. The cancer care team may include any or all of the following and others: primary care physicians, pathologists, pulmonologists, oncology specialists (medical oncologist, radiation oncologist), surgeons (including surgical specialists such as thoracic surgeons, neurosurgeons, etc.), nurses, oncology nurse specialists, and oncology social workers. Whether the team is linked formally or informally, there is usually one person who takes the job of coordinating the team. *See also* case manager, oncology.

cancer cell: a cell that divides and reproduces abnormally and has the potential to spread throughout the body, crowding out normal cells and tissue.

cancer-related fatigue: an unusual and persistent sense of tiredness that can occur with cancer or cancer treatments. It can be overwhelming, last a long time, and interfere with everyday life. Rest does not always relieve it.

carcinogen (car-SIN-o-jin): any substance that causes cancer or helps cancer grow. For example, tobacco smoke contains many carcinogens that greatly increase the risk of lung cancer.

carcinoid tumors (CAR-si-noid tumors): tumors that develop from neuroendocrine cells, usually in the digestive tract, lung, or ovary. The cancer cells from these tumors release certain hormones into the bloodstream. In about

10% of people, the hormone levels are high enough to cause facial flushing, wheezing, diarrhea, a fast heartbeat, and other symptoms throughout the body. Also known as carcinoids.

carcinoma (kahr-si-NO-muh): a malignant tumor that begins in the lining layer (epithelial cells) of organs. At least 80% of all cancers are carcinomas.

carcinoma in situ (kahr-si-NO-muh in SIGH-too): an early stage of cancer in which the tumor is confined to the organ where it first developed. The disease has not invaded other parts of the organ or spread to distant parts of the body. Most in situ carcinomas are highly curable. *See* in situ.

case manager: the member of a cancer care team, usually a nurse or oncology nurse specialist, who coordinates the patient's care throughout diagnosis, treatment, and recovery. The case manager is a new concept that provides a guide through the complex system of health care by helping cut through red tape, getting responses to questions, managing crises, and connecting the patient and family to needed resources.

cell: the basic unit of which all living things are made. Cells replace themselves by splitting and forming new cells (mitosis). The processes that control the formation of new cells and the death of old cells are disrupted in cancer. *See also* cell cycle.

cell cycle: the series of steps that a cell must go through to divide; some chemotherapy drugs act by interfering with the cell cycle.

chemotherapy (key-mo-THER-uh-pee): treatment with drugs to destroy cancer cells. Chemotherapy is often used, either alone or with surgery or radiation, to treat cancer that has spread or come back (recurred), or when there is a strong chance that it could recur. It is often called "chemo" for short.

chromosome (KROM-o-some): chromosomes carry the genes, the basic units of heredity. Humans have 23 pairs of chromosomes, one member of each pair from the mother, the other from the father. Each chromosome can contain hundreds or thousands of individual genes.

clinical trial: a research study to test new drugs or other treatments to compare current, standard treatments with others that may be better. Before a new treatment is used on people, it is studied in the lab. If lab studies suggest the treatment will work, the next step is to test its value for patients. These human studies are called clinical trials. The main questions the researchers want to answer are:

- Does this treatment work?
- Does it work better than what we're now using?
- What side effects does it cause?
- Do the benefits outweigh the risks?
- Which patients are most likely to find this treatment helpful?

See also randomized and control group.

complementary therapy: treatment used in addition to standard therapy. Some complementary therapies may help relieve certain symptoms of cancer, relieve side effects of standard cancer therapy, or improve a patient's sense of well-being. The American Cancer Society recommends that patients considering the use of any alternative or complementary therapy discuss this with their health care team, since many of these treatments are unproven and some can be harmful. *See also* alternative therapy, unproven therapy, and standard therapy.

computed tomography (computed tom-OG-ruh-fee): an imaging test in which many x-rays are taken from different angles of a part of the body. These images are combined by a computer to produce cross-sectional pictures of internal organs. Except for the injection of a dye (needed in some but not all cases), this is a painless procedure that can be done in an outpatient clinic. It is often referred to as a "CT" or "CAT" scan. *See also* CT–guided needle biopsy, spiral CT.

control group: in research or clinical trials, the group that does not receive the treatment being tested. The group may get a placebo or sham treatment, or it may receive standard therapy. Also called the comparison group. *See also* clinical trials, randomized.

CT–guided needle biopsy: a procedure that uses special x-rays to locate a mass, while the radiologist advances a biopsy needle toward it. The images are repeated until the doctor is sure the needle is in the tumor or mass. A biopsy is then taken from it to be looked at under the microscope. *See also* biopsy.

CT scan or CAT scan: *see* computed tomography.

cytology (sigh-TAHL-uh-jee): the branch of science that deals with the structure and function of cells. Also refers to tests to diagnose cancer and other diseases by examining cells under the microscope.

deoxyribonucleic acid (dee-ok-see-ri-bo-new-CLAY-ic acid): the genetic "blueprint" found in the nucleus of each cell. DNA holds genetic information on cell growth, division, and function. *See also* mutation; genome.

diagnosis: identifying a disease by its signs or symptoms, and by using imaging procedures and laboratory findings. The earlier a diagnosis of cancer is made, the better the chance for long-term survival.

dietary supplements: products, such as vitamins, minerals, or herbs, intended to improve health but not to diagnose, treat, cure, or prevent disease. Because dietary supplements are not considered "drugs," their manufacturers do not have to prove they are effective, or even safe. In many cases, studies have found that some do not contain what is advertised on the label, and some contain impurities or ingredients not listed.

DNA: *see* deoxyribonucleic acid and DNA repair.

DNA repair: the process of correcting the genetic mistakes that are made each time a cell divides. If the repair process does not go right, it can increase the chances of a person having some forms of cancer.

endoscopic esophageal ultrasound (en-do-SKOP-ik uh-sof-uh-JEE-uhl ultrasound) (EUS): a method in which a lighted, flexible scope is passed through the esophagus to permit ultrasound imaging from inside the esophagus. This method is useful for detecting large lymph nodes in the chest that may contain metastatic cancer.

external beam radiation therapy (EBRT): radiation that is focused from a source outside the body on the area affected by the cancer. It is much like getting a diagnostic x-ray, but for a longer time. *Compare to* brachytherapy, internal radiation.

false-positive: test result implying a condition exists when in fact it does not.

fatigue (fuh-TEEG): a common symptom during cancer treatment, a bone-weary exhaustion that doesn't get better with rest. For some, this can last for some time after treatment. *See also* cancer-related fatigue.

first-degree relative: a first-degree relative is defined as a parent, sibling, or child.

five (5)-year survival rate: the percentage of people with a given cancer who are expected to survive 5 years or longer after diagnosis. Five-year survival rates are based on the most recent information available, but they may include information from patients treated several years earlier. These numbers do not take into account advances in treatment that have often occurred. They are not helpful in predicting an individual case. They only paint a very general picture of how people in the past have done with the same type of cancer. *See also* relative 5-year survival rate, survival rate.

gene: a segment of DNA that contains information on hereditary characteristics such as hair color, eye color, and height, as well as susceptibility to certain diseases. *See also* deoxyribonucleic acid.

gene therapy: the insertion of genes into an individual's body to treat disease, in particular hereditary diseases. *See also* gene, and genome.

genome (JEE-nome): the total DNA in a single cell, representing all of the genetic information of the organism.

grade: the grade of a cancer reflects how abnormal it looks under the microscope. There are several grading systems for different types of cancers. Each grading system divides cancer into those with the greatest abnormality, the least abnormality, and those in between.

Grading is done by a pathologist who examines the tissue from the biopsy. It is important because cancers with more abnormal-appearing cells tend to grow and spread more quickly and have a worse prognosis (outlook). *See also* histology.

high risk: when the chance of developing cancer is greater than that normally seen in the general population. People may be at high risk from many factors, including heredity (such as a family history of breast cancer), personal habits (such as smoking), or the environment (such as overexposure to sunlight).

histology (hiss-TAH-luh-jee): how cells or tissues look when studied under a microscope. The histologic examination is done by a pathologist. *See also* pathologist.

Hodgkin disease: an often curable type of cancer that affects the lymphatic system. Named for the doctor who first identified it; previously called Hodgkin's disease.

home health nurse: a nurse who gives medications in the home, teaches patients how to care for themselves at home, and assesses their condition to see if further medical attention is needed.

hormone: a chemical substance released into the body by the endocrine glands such as the thyroid, adrenal, or ovaries. Hormones travel through the bloodstream and set in motion various body functions. Testosterone and estrogen are examples of male and female hormones.

hospice: a special kind of care for people in the final phase of illness, their families, and their caregivers. The care may take place in the patient's home or in a homelike facility. *See also* home health nurse.

imaging test: a method used to produce pictures of internal body structures. Some imaging tests used to help diagnose or stage cancer are x-rays, CT scans, magnetic resonance imaging (MRI), and ultrasound.

immune system: the complex system by which the body resists infection by germs such as bacteria or viruses and rejects transplanted tissues or organs. The immune system may also help the body fight some cancers. *See also* immunology, immunosuppression.

immunology (im-yuh-NAHL-uh-jee): study of how the body resists infection and certain other diseases. Knowledge gained in this field is important to those cancer treatments based on the principles of immunology.

immunosuppression (im-mune-no-suh-PREH-shun): a state in which the ability of the body's immune system to respond is decreased. This condition may be present at birth, or it may be caused by certain infections (such as human immunodeficiency virus or HIV), or by certain cancer therapies, such as chemotherapy, radiation, and bone marrow transplantation.

immunotherapy (im-mune-no-THER-uh-pee): treatments that promote or support the body's immune system response to a disease such as cancer.

informed consent: a legal document that explains a course of treatment, the risks, benefits, and possible alternatives; the process by which patients agree to treatment.

in situ (in SIGH-too): in place; localized and confined to one area. A very early stage of cancer.

internal radiation: treatment involving implantation of a radioactive substance; *see* brachytherapy. *Compare to* external beam radiation therapy.

intravenous (in-tra-VEEN-us) (IV): a method of supplying fluids and medications using a needle or a thin tube inserted in a vein (called a catheter).

large-cell undifferentiated carcinoma (large-cell undifferentiated kahr-si-NO-muh): cancer that may appear in any part of the lung. The cells are large and look abnormal when viewed under a microscope. They tend to grow and spread quickly.

lobectomy (lob-BEK-to-me): surgery to remove a lobe of an organ—usually the lung.

lymphatic system: the tissues and organs (including lymph nodes, spleen, thymus, and bone marrow) that produce and store lymphocytes (cells that fight infection) and the channels that carry the lymph fluid. The entire lymphatic system is an important part of the body's immune system. Invasive cancers sometimes penetrate the lymphatic vessels (channels) and spread (metastasize) to lymph nodes.

lymph nodes: small bean-shaped collections of immune system tissue found along lymphatic vessels. They remove waste, germs, and other harmful substances from lymph (a colorless fluid that bathes body tissues). They help fight infections and have a role in fighting cancer, though sometimes cancer spreads through them. *See also* lymphatic system.

magnetic resonance imaging (MRI): a method of taking pictures of the inside of the body. Instead of using x-rays, MRI uses a powerful magnet to send radio waves through the body. The images appear on a computer screen as well as on film. Like x-rays, the procedure is physically painless, but some people may feel confined inside the MRI machine.

malignant (muh-LIG-nant) tumor: a mass of cancer cells that may invade surrounding tissues or spread (metastasize) to distant areas of the body. *See also* tumor, metastasis.

mediastinoscopy (me-dee-uh-stine-AHS-ko-pee): examination of the chest cavity using a lighted tube inserted under the chest bone (sternum). This allows the doctor to see the lymph nodes in this area and remove samples to check for cancer.

mediastinotomy (me-dee-uh-stine-AH-to-mee): a procedure in which the doctor makes an incision into the mediastinum (defined below).

mediastinum (me-dee-uh-STI-nuhm): the space in the chest cavity behind the chest bone (sternum) and between the 2 lungs.

metastasis (meh-TAS-teh-sis): cancer cells that have spread to one or more sites elsewhere in the body, often by way of the lymph system or bloodstream. Regional metastasis is cancer that has spread to the lymph nodes, tissues, or organs close to the primary site. Distant metastasis is cancer that has spread to organs or tissues that are farther away (such as when prostate cancer spreads to the bones, lungs, or liver).The plural of this word is metastases. *See also* primary site, lymph nodes, micrometastases, regional involvement.

metastasize (meh-TAS-tuh-size): the spread of cancer cells to one or more sites elsewhere in the body, often by way of the lymphatic system or bloodstream. *See also* metastasis, lymphatic system.

metastatic (met-uh-STAT-ick): a way to describe cancer that has spread from the primary site (where it started) to other structures or organs, nearby or far away (distant). *See also* primary site, metastasis, micrometastases.

micrometastases (mike-row-muh-TAS-tuh-seez): the spread of cancer cells in groups so small that they can only be seen under a microscope.

MRI: *see* magnetic resonance imaging.

mutation: a change in the DNA of a cell. Most mutations do not produce cancer, and a few may even be helpful. However, all types of cancer are thought to be due to mutations that damage a cell's DNA. Some cancer-related mutations can be inherited, which means that the person is born with the mutated DNA in all the body's cells. However, most mutations happen after the person is born, and are called somatic mutations. This type of mutation happens in one cell at a time, and only affects cells that arise from the single mutated cell. *See also* DNA.

needle aspiration: a type of needle biopsy. Removal of fluid from a cyst or cells from a tumor. In this procedure, a needle is used to reach the cyst or tumor, and with suction, draw up (aspirate) samples for examination under a microscope. If the needle is thin, the procedure is called a fine needle aspiration or FNA. *See also* biopsy, needle biopsy.

needle biopsy: removal of fluid, cells, or tissue with a needle for examination under a microscope. There are 2 types: fine needle aspiration (FNA) and core biopsy. FNA uses a thin needle to draw up (aspirate) fluid or small tissue fragments from a cyst or tumor. A core needle biopsy uses a thicker needle to remove a cylindrical sample of tissue from a tumor.

oncogenes (ON-ko-genes): genes that promote cell growth and multiplication. These genes are normally present in all cells. But oncogenes may undergo changes that activate them, causing cells to grow too quickly and form tumors. *Compare to* tumor suppressor genes.

oncology (on-CALL-o-jee): the branch of medicine concerned with the diagnosis and treatment of cancer.

p53: a protein that is mutated in more than 50% of tumors. The normal (not mutated) form of p53 keeps the cell from entering the cell division cycle. It has also been found to bring about cell death (apoptosis) after DNA damage. *See also* mutation.

palliative treatment (PAL-e-uh-tive TREET-muhnt): treatment that relieves symptoms, such as pain, but is not expected to cure the disease. Its main purpose is to improve the patient's quality of life. Sometimes chemotherapy and radiation are used in this way.

pathologist (path-AHL-o-jist): a doctor who specializes in diagnosis and classification of diseases by lab tests such as examining cells under a microscope. The pathologist determines whether a tumor is benign or cancerous, and if cancerous the exact cell type and grade. *See also* cytology.

performance status: A general measurement of health or a term used to describe a cancer patient's general well-being or quality of life. This measure is used to determine whether a patient can receive chemotherapy, whether dose adjustment is necessary, and as a measure for the amount of supportive care needed.

PET scan: *see* positron emission tomography.

photodynamic therapy (foe-toe-die-NAM-ick therapy) (PDT): a treatment sometimes used for cancers of the skin, esophagus, lung, or bladder. PDT begins with the injection of a nontoxic chemical into the blood. This chemical is attracted to cancer cells and is allowed to collect in the tumor for a few days. A special type of laser light is then focused on the cancer. This light causes the chemical to change so that it can kill cancer cells. The advantage of PDT is that it can kill cancer cells with very little harm to normal cells.

pleura (PLOO-ruh): the membrane around the lungs and lining of the chest cavity.

pleurodesis (ploo-row-DEE-sis): injection of a agent between the layers of the pleura that causes them to fuse them together to seal off leaks. This procedure helps prevent fluid or air from building up in the pleural cavity.

pneumonectomy (new-mo-NEK-to-me): surgery to remove an entire lung.

positron emission tomography (PAHS-uh trahn ee-MISH-uhn tom-AGH-ruh-fee) (PET): a PET scan creates an image of the body after the injection of a very low dose of radioactive sugar (glucose). The scan computes the rate at which the tumor is using the sugar. In general, cancer cells use large amounts of the sugar. PET scans look at the whole body and are especially useful in taking images of the brain. They are becoming more widely used to find the spread of cancer of the breast, colon, rectum, ovary, or lung. PET scans may also be used to see how well the tumor is responding to treatment.

precancerous: *see* premalignant.

premalignant: changes in cells that may, but do not always, become cancer. Also called precancerous.

prevention: the reduction of cancer risk by eliminating or reducing contact with carcinogenic agents. A change in lifestyle, such as quitting smoking, for example, reduces the risk of lung and other cancers.

primary site: the place where cancer begins. Primary cancer is usually named after the organ in which it starts. For example, cancer that starts in the breast is always breast cancer even if it spreads (metastasizes) to other organs, such as bones or lungs.

prognosis (prog-NO-sis): a prediction of the course of disease; the outlook for the chances of survival.

quality of life: overall enjoyment of life, which includes a person's sense of well-being and ability to do the things that are important to him or her.

radiation dose: the amount of radiation an object (such as human tissue) receives. There are several units used to describe radiation doses:

> **rad ("radiation absorbed dose"):** a basic unit of the amount of radiation transferred to an object. This measurement does not take into account the type of radiation, which can influence the effect on different body tissues. The rad has largely been replaced by the gray (see next).

> **gray (Gy):** the newer, international unit of measurement of radiation transfer. One gray equals 100 rads. (Therefore, one rad equals one centigray [cGy].)

rem ("roentgen equivalent man"): a basic unit of radiation exposure, which is based on both the dose and the type of radiation. Because of this, it is more commonly used to describe radiation exposure than is the rad. Often reported in units of millirem (mrem), which is one-thousandth of a rem. The rem is sometimes replaced by the sievert (see next).

sievert (Sv): the newer, international unit of measurement of radiation exposure. One sievert equals 100 rem. Often reported in millisieverts (mSv), which are thousandths of a sievert (or about $1/10$ of a rem).

radiation therapy: treatment with high-energy rays (such as x-rays) to kill or shrink cancer cells. The radiation may come from outside of the body (external radiation) or from radioactive materials placed directly in the tumor (brachytherapy or internal radiation). Radiation therapy may be used as the main treatment for a cancer, to reduce the size of a cancer before surgery, or to destroy any remaining cancer cells after surgery. In advanced cancer cases, it may also be used as palliative treatment. *See also* external beam radiation therapy, brachytherapy, palliative treatment, radiation dose.

randomized or randomization: a process used in clinical trials that uses chance to assign participants to different groups that compare treatments. Randomization means that each person has an equal chance of being in the treatment and comparison groups. This helps reduce the chance of bias in the results that might happen, if, for example, the healthiest people all were assigned to a particular treatment group. *See also* control group, clinical trials.

recurrence: the return of cancer after treatment. Local recurrence means that the cancer has come back at the same place as the original cancer. Regional recurrence means that the cancer has come back after treatment near the primary site. Distant recurrence is when cancer metastasizes after treatment to distant organs or tissues. *See also* primary site, metastasis, metastasize.

regimen (REH-juh-men): a strict, regulated plan (such as diet, exercise, or medication schedule) designed to reach certain goals. In cancer treatment, a plan to treat cancer.

regional involvement or regional spread: the spread of cancer from its original site to nearby areas such as lymph nodes, but not to distant sites. *See also* metastasis.

relapse: reappearance of cancer after a disease-free period. *See* recurrence.

relative 5-year survival rate: the percentage of people with a certain cancer who have not died from it within 5 years. This number is different from the 5-year survival rate in that the relative 5-year survival rate does not include people who have died from unrelated causes. *See also* 5-year survival rate and survival rate.

remission: complete or partial disappearance of the signs and symptoms of cancer in response to treatment; the period during which a disease is under control. A remission may not be a cure.

resection: surgery to remove part or all of an organ or other structure.

risk factor: anything that is related to a person's chance of getting a disease such as cancer. Different cancers have different risk factors. For example, unprotected exposure to strong sunlight is a risk factor for skin cancer; smoking is a risk factor for lung, mouth, larynx, and other cancers. Some risk factors, such as smoking, can be controlled. Others, like a person's age, can't be changed.

scan: a study using either x-rays or radioactive isotopes to produce images of internal body organs.

screening: the search for disease, such as cancer, in people without symptoms. For example, screening measures for prostate cancer include digital rectal examination and the PSA blood test; for breast cancer, mammograms and clinical breast exams. Screening may refer to coordinated programs in large groups of people.

segmentectomy: removal of part of a lobe (section) of the lung. Also known as wedge resection.

side effects: unwanted effects of treatment such as hair loss caused by chemotherapy, and fatigue caused by radiation therapy.

sign: an observable physical change caused by an illness. *Compare to* symptom.

spiral CT: a special scanner that takes cross-sectional pictures around the body. *See also* computed tomography.

sputum cytology (SPU-tum sigh-TAHL-uh-gee): a study of phlegm cells under a microscope to see whether they are normal or not.

squamous cell carcinoma (SKWAY-mus cell kahr-si-NO-muh): cancer that begins in the non-glandular cells, for example, the skin.

staging: the process of finding out whether cancer has spread and if so, how far; that is, to learn the stage of the cancer. The AJCC/TNM system is used for staging non–small cell lung cancer.

The TNM system gives 3 key pieces of information:

T refers to the size of the tumor

N describes how far the cancer has spread to nearby lymph nodes

M shows whether the cancer has spread (metastasized) to other organs of the body

Letters or numbers after the T, N, and M give more details about each of these factors. To make this information clearer, the TNM descriptions can be grouped together into a simpler set of stages, labeled with Roman numerals (usually from I to IV). In general, the lower the number, the less the cancer has spread. A higher number means a more serious cancer.

The 2 types of staging are:

clinical staging: an estimate of the extent of cancer based on physical exam, biopsy results, and imaging tests.

pathologic staging: an estimate of the extent of cancer by direct study of the samples removed during surgery.

See also grade.

standard therapy: standard treatment: *see* therapy.

survival rate: the percentage of people still alive within a certain period of time after diagnosis or treatment. For cancer, a 5-year survival rate is often given. This does not mean that people can't live more than 5 years, or that those who live for 5 years are necessarily permanently cured. *See also* relative 5-year survival rate.

symptom: a change in the body caused by an illness, as described by the person experiencing it. *Compare to* sign.

therapy: any of the measures taken to treat a disease. *See also* alternative therapy, complementary therapy, unproven therapy, and standard therapy.

thoracentesis (thor-uh-sen-TEE-sis): a procedure during which the skin is numbed and a needle is placed between the ribs to drain fluid that surrounds the lung. The fluid is checked under a microscope to look for cancer cells. Fluid buildup can prevent the lungs from filling with air, so thoracentesis can help the patient breathe better and may be repeated as needed.

thoracoscopy (thor-uh-KAH-skuh-pee): a procedure during which small incisions are made in the chest to permit insertion of surgical tools such as the thoracoscope— a long tube with a magnifying glass and light on the end. This procedure permits the doctor to see cancer deposits and remove tissues to be examined.

tissue: a collection of cells, united to perform a particular function.

TNM staging system: *see* staging.

trachea (TRAY-key-uh): the "windpipe." The trachea connects the larynx (voice box) with the bronchi and serves as the main passage for air into the lungs.

transtracheal fine needle aspiration (trans-TRAY-kee-uhl fine needle aspiration): a procedure by which a thin needle is inserted into the wall of the trachea and guided by bronchoscopy to sample nearby lymph nodes. This method is used to detect cancerous cells and determine whether cancer has spread.

tumor: an abnormal lump or mass of tissue. Tumors can be benign (non-cancerous) or malignant (cancerous).

tumor suppressor genes: genes that slow down cell division or cause cells to die at the appropriate time. Alterations of these genes can lead to too much cell growth and development of cancer.

ultrasound: an imaging method in which high-frequency sound waves are used to outline a part of the body. The sound wave echoes are picked up and displayed on a television screen. Also called ultrasonography.

unproven therapy: any therapy that has not been scientifically tested and approved.

x-ray: one form of radiation that can be used at low levels to produce an image of the body on film or at high levels to destroy cancer cells.

Index

INFORMATION FOR PEOPLE WITH CANCER

Site-Specific

9538.00   A Breast Cancer Journey, Second Edition

9658.00   ACS's Complete Guide to Colorectal Cancer

9652.00   ACS's Complete Guide to Prostate Cancer

9661.00   QuickFACTS™ Colon Cancer

9660.00   QuickFACTS™ Prostate Cancer

Symptom Management

9637.00   ACS's Guide to Pain Control, Revised Edition

9633.00   Eating Well, Staying Well During and After Cancer

9657.01   Lymphedema: Understanding and Managing Lymphedema After Cancer Treatment

Praise for **QuickFACTS™ Lung Cancer**, and **QuickFACTS™ Advanced Cancer**: *"The ACS has achieved its goal of providing overviews that tackle need-to-know issues and supply references for additional follow-up information as desired. Recommended."* —Library Journal

Praise for **Lymphedema**: *"Written in a supportive and accessible voice, the book [Lymphedema] will be most useful to those who have been touched by lymphedema and who are seeking comprehensive and authoritative coverage of their concerns. Recommended for public and consumer health libraries."* —Library Journal

QuickFACTS **Lung Cancer**

SUPPORT FOR FAMILIES AND CAREGIVERS

9435.00 Cancer in the Family (Helping Children
Cope with a Parent's Illness)

4660.00 Cancer Support Groups (A Guide
for Facilitators)

9527.00 Caregiving (A Step-by-Step Resource for
Caring for the Person with Cancer At Home,
Revised Edition)

9512.00 Couples Confronting Cancer (Keeping Your
Relationship Strong)

9651.00 When the Focus Is on Care
(Palliative Care and Cancer)

Praise for **Caregiving**: *"A thorough and accessible resource."*
—Former First Lady Rosalynn Carter,
Author, *Helping Yourself Help Others*

*"Chock-full of sensible and reassuring information, easily
accessible to the average reader. Good glossary and extensive
resource section included. Recommended."* —Library Journal

*"...Designed for caregivers but is equally informative for the
patient. Well-organized."* —Bookpage

HELP FOR CHILDREN

9513.00 Because...Someone I Love Has Cancer (Kids'
Activity Book)

9496.00 Our Mom Has Cancer (hard cover)

9457.00 Our Mom Has Cancer (paperback)

Praise for **Our Mom Has Cancer**: *"I needed a way to let
my children know what they could expect as far as my
therapy, and let them know what might happen emotionally.
...Excellent, and I would recommend it to any parent who has
been diagnosed..."* —A mom from Cedar Rapids, Iowa

CANCER INFORMATION

9632.00	Cancer: What Causes It, What Doesn't
9505.00	Coming to Terms with Cancer (A Glossary of Cancer-Related Terms)
9449.02	Informed Decisions, Second Edition
9670.00	The Cancer Atlas (English)
9671.00	The Cancer Atlas (Spanish)
9672.00	The Cancer Atlas (French)
9673.00	The Cancer Atlas (Chinese)
9674.00	The Tobacco Atlas, Second Edition (English)
9675.00	The Tobacco Atlas, Second Edition (Spanish)
9676.00	The Tobacco Atlas, Second Edition (French)
9677.00	The Tobacco Atlas, Second Edition (Chinese)

INSPIRATIONAL SURVIVOR STORIES

9540.00   I Can Survive (Illustrated)

9510.00   Angels & Monsters (A child's eye view of cancer)

9463.00   Crossing Divides (A Couple's Story of Cancer, Hope and Hiking Montana's Continental Divide)

Praise for **Angels & Monsters**: *"Stunningly beautiful and thought-provoking…Sensitive, insightful, unique and thoroughly "kid-friendly." Highly recommended reading for any child [and parent] having to cope with cancer, and would make a welcome and valued addition to any school or community library collection."* —Midwest Book Review

Praise for **Crossing Divides**: *"Every life has its mountains to climb. Read on and find the inspiration to reach your summit."* —Bernie Siegel, MD

"The challenges of confronting the dangers and frustrations of the wilderness become a metaphor in this fascinating book for facing the challenges of a cancer illness. …Love of life and love of nature are fused into a remarkable human experience that ensures the reader will find new meaning in juxtaposition with illness." —Jimmie C. Holland, MD, Chair, Department of Psychiatry & Behavorial Sciences, Memorial Sloan-Kettering Cancer Center

TOOLS FOR THE HEALTH CONSCIOUS

9403.01	ACS's Healthy Eating Cookbook, Third Edition
9437.00	Celebrate! (Healthy Entertaining for Any Occasion)
9471.00	Good For You! (Reducing Your Risk of Developing Cancer)
9511.00	Kicking Butts (Quit Smoking and Take Charge of Your Health)

HEALTHY BOOKS FOR CHILDREN

9401.00	Kids' First Cookbook (Delicious-Nutritious Treats to Make Yourself!)
9100.00	Healthy Me (A Read-along Coloring & Activity Book)
2027.27	National Health Education Standards: Achieving Excellence, Second Edition

Praise for **Kids' First Cookbook**: *"A cookbook with a contemporary look filled with nutrition information. The uncluttered....layout is pleasing and employs colored type, drawings, and helpful photographs. A solid effort that will encourage healthy eating habits."* —School Library Journal